WARRIOR PRINCESS

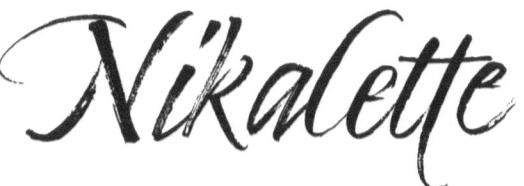

AND HER BATTLE AGAINST EPILEPSY

LILIA SIMENTAL

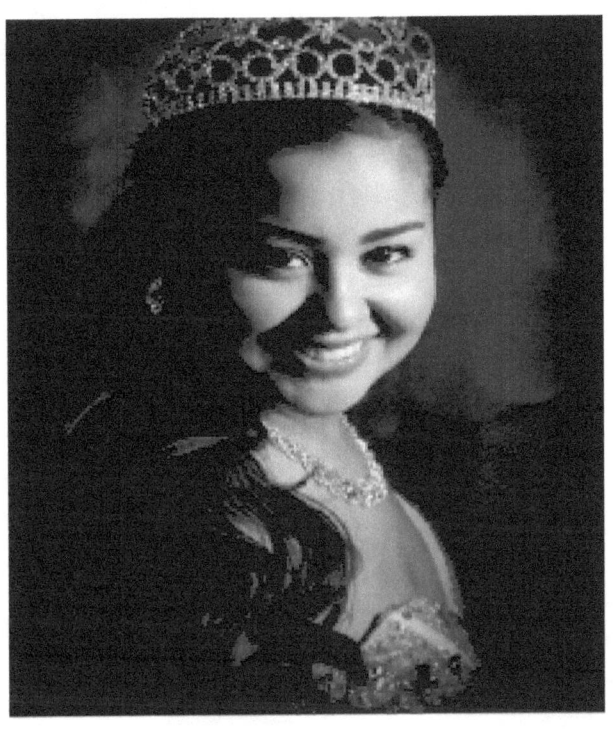

Warrior Princess Nikalette And Her Battle Against Epilepsy

*A Biography to honor Nikalette Simental-Rivera
our Yabucoa Puerto Rican Princess
2017-2018*

Dedication

I am Lilia Simental, the grandmother of Nikalette. I want to dedicate this book to God's presence in our lives. Thank God for the fantastic seventeen years Nikalette Yliana Simental-Rivera, our Warrior Princess, an extraordinary girl, was present in our lives.

This story will describe my granddaughter Nikalette's life and how she impacted others with her warm, lovely, compassionate, and energetic personality. She helped others in so many ways during her short life. Nikalette suffered from nocturnal tonic-clonic (grand mal) seizures. This condition led to her sudden, unexpected death.

In addition, I dedicate this book to all people who have epilepsy, their families, caregivers, and other loved ones, and the community of Aurora, Illinois, who helped me tremendously. I also include here Nikalette's most memorable experiences and her poems, as well as letters written posthumously to Nikalette. They all add vivid testimonial notes to this book that aims to share Nikalette's life experience, and I hope they will paint a clear picture for you as the reader.

This book aims to improve epilepsy knowledge and to provide the skills to prevent or limit serious injuries or possibly sudden death, as happened to Nikalette. It also presents current research data for grieving in a healthy manner with God's presence, plus my experience as a faithful registered nurse.

Finally, this book is dedicated to honor Nikalette's overall life and presents a biography of a beautiful and humble adolescent who did a lot in her short time with us. She was an actual warrior princess who battled against epilepsy and so many other difficulties in her life and the lives of others. Although she battled against epilepsy every day, Nikalette still lived her life to its fullest potential by doing what she wanted to do as a fine Catholic Christian girl.

Contents

Foreword

I am honored to remark upon this book. I have worked closely with the author, Lilia Simental, for more than thirty years at Rush University Medical Center in Chicago Illinois. Lilia is a loving mother; beloved, dedicated grandmother; respected nurse manager; and compassionate registered nurse. Lilia is among the elite in *Who's Who in American Nursing* and the recipient of multiple nursing awards. She is a leader, an outstanding mentor, and a superior clinical nurse in rehabilitation, geriatrics, medical, surgical, and community health nursing.

This biography pays tribute to Lilia's seventeen-year-old granddaughter, Nikalette, who tragically died from epilepsy. Those afflicted with epilepsy experience a chronic illness, and those who are affected should take measures to shield themselves from bullying, uncomfortable embarrassment, and painful ridicule. This biography illuminates the struggles of Nikalette and her family. Those with epilepsy and their families may gain strength from the common ground in knowing they are not alone. In Nikalette's abbreviated life, she became a remarkable high school leader, mentor to her peers, and role model for high moral and ethical values. Being named

Miss Yabucoa Puerto Rican Princess was the highlight of her young life. Nikalette was a beautiful teen, mature beyond her years. Her life story will hopefully inspire others, especially you, the reader. The family's strong faith and spirituality have supported them through Nikalette's childhood diagnosis and adolescence. During life and even after her death, Nikalette taught us that a spiritual foundation can guide us on a righteous path to reach our goals. When we elevate others to believe in themselves, they can achieve the extraordinary through perseverance and a warm, compassionate heart.

Margaret Waszkiewicz, MS RN CRRN, CNA-BC. Award -Winning nursing leader, clinician, and magnet nursing speaker.

Introduction

"The just have perished, but no one takes it to heart; the steadfast are swept away, while no one understands. Yet the just are taken away from the presence of evil, and enter into peace; they rest upon their couches, the sincere, who walk in integrity."
- Isaiah 57:1–2

I am cheerful and passionately believe that God took Nikalette to heaven early in her life to avoid any more suffering and pain from epilepsy, the chronic illness that she suffered with for more than eight years. This true-life story illustrates our strong faith in God, which is still helping our family and friends to cope with the sudden loss of Nikalette.

Our faith in God has been a significant asset in enhancing our trust in Jesus Christ, uniting us as family, friends, and the community of Aurora, Illinois, a suburb of Chicago. This tragedy has brought about a difficult time of grief. We have experienced unbearable pain from the death of Miss Puerto Rican Yabucoa's first princess for 2017–2018, Nikalette Yliana Simental-Rivera.

I know that Nikalette wanted to share her life experiences. She was a dynamic, intelligent, sweet young lady who loved people, a person that we should all emulate. She was highly spiritual, productive, and achieved many goals at a young age while she battled epilepsy.

CHAPTER 1

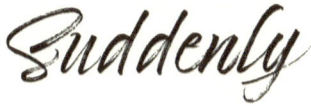

My dear, loving granddaughter died suddenly in her sleep, after or during a seizure, at the age of seventeen, on May 10, 2018. I am constantly thinking of Nikalette's tragic end. The suffering from the loss of her affected me to the point that I could not return to work as a nurse in any clinical setting, a job that is my passion. I had worked full time for more than thirty years at Rush University Medical Center in Chicago, Illinois. I take this opportunity to ask God and Nikalette for forgiveness that I did not save her life.

My granddaughter motivated me to write this book. I just want to honor the life of Nikalette. It was a challenging, traumatic experience, on top of her loss's unbearable pain and grief. The pain leads me continuously to think of what I could have done differently to save her. I feel that this experience may be able to help others who are facing a loss with such a traumatic event. I think that writing and doing an extensive review of the literature on epilepsy and grief is part of my therapy to relieve my emotional pain and to heal my soul, but at same time I can help others who are in similar conditions than me.

On May 10, I felt sick the second I woke up that morning. I had flu-like symptoms. I had aches and pains in my body and slight chest congestion. I still got up early and did my best to get my grandkids ready for school. I hydrated myself, took Tylenol for my headache, and continued moving on with my daily routine. I prepared breakfast, lunch, and dinner. I took Nikalette to school at 7:30 AM after our morning prayers. Then I returned at 3 PM to pick her up from Aurora West High School.

My daughter Sandy, Nikalette's mother, was looking to buy a house for herself and her four children. They lived in my home with me and my husband temporarily for approximately three years. My granddaughter Nikalette said to me that morning, "Today I will go with you and help look for a house for my mom and my family." Nikalette had promised her mom she would go with me to see the house. We went to the small town of Montgomery, Illinois, and saw a house from the inside and the outside. People were still living in it and their dogs were locked up in the basement. But Nikalette went directly to the dogs and played with them for a few moments. She looked happy playing with them. Then she was talking on the phone with her friend Monica, one of her best friends, telling her about the house we visited. She said,

"We might get a home in Montgomery, Illinois," meaning she would possibly have to attend Oswego High School.

My daughter went to work around 6 PM. Nikalette and Sean, her younger brother, ate dinner, and both went to their bedroom on the second floor to do homework. I took Angelina, her younger sister, to her friend's house to do a school project. Sam Anthony, Nikalette's older brother, came home from his job, ate dinner, and went to the gym around 8:30 PM. My husband ate a late dinner with me around 9:15 PM, while Nikalette went upstairs to take a shower. Then my husband told me he would take his shower in the basement after he finished eating. I sat in the family room taking a break from the busy day, since I was still not feeling well from the morning. I took Tylenol again to reduce the body aches. Sean, Nikalette's youngest brother, went with his friend from school to play basketball. Overall, each family member had their own activity going on, and the house was not as busy as usual.

I sent a text message to Nikalette to check in. She did not answer me, which was very unusual. I did feel a sharp pain in my chest. I became very apprehensive and nervous at the same time. It was a bizarre feeling, on top of the congestion and arthritic pains in my back. I panicked when she did not answer her phone; Nikalette always responded to my texts immediately. I ran to her room on the second floor, but I did not think to take my phone with me.

That night was the worst time in my life. This horrific experience will forever be in my mind. I found Nikalette in her bed lying on her stomach, prone position, unconscious with no breathing, and her pupils fix and were noticeably dilated. My husband was still taking a shower and no one else was around. So, I had no choice but to try to save Nikalette's life on my own. I brought her to the floor and started mouth-to-mouth resuscitation and compressions on her chest. (Compressions are more effective on the floor, which serves as a firm surface.) I performed cardiopulmonary resuscitation for an extended period; it was a stressful time. The stress and pressure increase tremendously when you are doing CPR on a loved one, or any other person, all by yourself. You get exhausted quickly. I was in shock for an extended period, and I lost track of time.

I did everything correctly, but Nikalette remained unconscious, not responding to CPR. I did not know how much longer it would take to continue trying to resuscitate her. My husband finally came up from the basement and called 911. This tragedy was a life and death situation, extremely stressful, and every second counted. Three paramedics entered our home and started asking us many questions while taking over CPR. They asked me how long I had done the CPR. I was unsure of the time but responded with an estimate. One of the paramedics wanted to clarify: "You did thirty minutes?" I barely answered yes. I was unsure because I did not keep track. I was exhausted and ready to pass out. My brain had difficulty remembering the events before and during this tragic situation minute by minute. They asked my husband and me to leave the bedroom, which we did, and I went to the adjacent room with one of the paramedics. The other two paramedics worked with Nikalette for ten to fifteen minutes. I regret not staying in the room to assist the paramedics; when I saw them, I was relieved but also was not myself. I was in shock and ready to pass out from the effects of this challenging and stressful situation. I felt relief that they could help us with Nikalette, but I was still worried that she was not responding to any stimuli.

Then I heard one of the paramedics say, "She is gone; we need to call the coroner." The paramedics called the coroner and also called Nikalette's mom. She worked in critical medical care at Loyola Medical Center, forty-five minutes away from our home. She is a Certified Respiratory Therapist and was scheduled to work the night shift. I could not believe what I had just heard; I just wanted to die myself. I felt I should have been the one to go to heaven instead, since I have lived a full life. My husband and I were closer than she was to going with our Lord since we were both older and had just retired.

The death of my lovely granddaughter made me numb and empty, left me in disbelief and shock. I asked myself, "WHY? WHY? Why was I not able to save her life?" I cried endlessly. My husband was also in shock. We both were trying to take a deep breath. Angelina was dropped off by her friend's mom shortly after her sister's death. We tried to console her the best that we could. That night, I tried to compose myself by asking God to give me the strength, as He always did in the past, to assist others. We prayed to God to help us through this catastrophic event.

I thought that the paramedics would take Nikalette to the hospital and that she would be OK. We had had a similar situation in the past, and they had taken her to the hospital due to a prolonged seizure. But this time was different.

Shortly after the paramedics had arrived, Sean and Anthony returned home from their baseball and gym activities. They were upset and crying loudly and started to call family and friends. I hugged all my grandchildren and my husband. I noticed my husband had tremors and was extremely anxious. We all cried and cried together for hours but were still in shock. My house was full of people, with family and friends immediately praying for and consoling us. Everyone asked me multiple questions, several of them related to seizure activity. I felt like I was going to faint.

The coroner came to take Nikalette to perform an autopsy. The coroner asked me multiple questions. My head was in a fog. I was trying to comprehend everything, but it was also exhausting. This tragic event was so sudden, extremely painful, and hard for me to assimilate. It did not make any sense. One minute you are fine; the next minute you are not. After 11 PM, the coroner called Rev. Monsignor Father Robert Willhite from St. Joseph Church, a retired pastor who has been with our family for more than forty-six years, to inform him of Nikalette's death. He also called Father Gerardo Manuel Gomez Reza, who prayed and did the Mass for us in the morning. Both of them said they could not come right away but began praying for us. Both priests, Father Gerardo Manuel and Father Robert, provided emotional and spiritual support for us. We were incredibly appreciative of their time. Without them, we do not know how we could have faced this painful experience.

That night after 11:15 PM, I called Father Gerardo Manuel Gomez Reza from St. Rita Church myself. He was a young priest, a very dedicated priest. He knew Nikalette well and had prepared her for multiple religious events, such as her Quinceañera and the Sacrament of her Confirmation. She always went to Father Manuel for confessions. Nikalette had a good rapport with Father Manuel Gomez. He subsequently did prayers for her funeral wake at the Daleiden Funeral Home in Aurora, Illinois, and said her funeral Mass and graveside service. We felt remarkably close to Father Manuel. Unfortunately, we lost him on December 26, 2019, due to cancer, and he is now with Nikalette in heaven.

I did not want to go back into Nikalette's room that night, but a lot of her classmates did. They went into her room every time they were in my house, and they touched her clothes, cried, and prayed. At times we would cry together. But everything happened so fast that we were all in shock and denial. It was so sudden and excruciating that our minds were foggy and unable to think clearly. We did not sleep much for several days and weeks as we planned for the funeral services, waiting for the rest of our family to arrive. Almost a week later, several came from Mexico, from Texas, from Tampa, Florida, and from other places. They also provided a lot of emotional, spiritual support and love to all of us. They brought food and flowers. We all prayed together. Several times Monsignor Robert Willhite and other church leaders came too. We all prayed for the rosary at 5 PM for nine days. Those days of prayers were the only thing that consoled me, my family, and the others who joined our prayers.

After we buried Nikalette, I did not want to wake up anymore if I could not see her smile. Her room, right next to mine, now was empty. It was very sad and painful.

Since May 10, 2018, the day that shattered our hearts into pieces, our emotions have been ongoing. Nothing could relieve my pain, well, except when I attended church for daily Mass, prayed the rosary, and gave everything to the Lord. It was beneficial for my family and me to spend a long time at church praying.

Later we found out from her classmates that Nikalette had had a lot of stress during that day, May 10, 2018. She took two tests and gave a presentation in Spanish. One of Nikalette's close friends told her that her boyfriend was seen with another girl. She also found out one of her close uncles, Jose ()Pucho Rivera, her father's brother, had had an accident. Nikalette's uncle was like a father figure to her. Overall, accumulated stress was one of the main causes of seizures for Nikalette.

This tragedy instantly changed my life. Not only did it negatively affect me, but it also negatively affected the rest of Nikalette's family, her classmates, her friends, and the whole town of Aurora. The sudden loss of my granddaughter did not allow me to say good-bye to Nikalette and her unfinished dreams, her high school, her desire to go to medical school and to help other people with epilepsy. She had wanted to study neurology in the future and to bring people closer to our Lord.

Nikalette's room is intact. She always loved to keep her room clean. Her decorations are in bright colors such as pink, purple, and blue. Her drapes are pink, and the bedspread is blue and pink—very colorful. Her furniture is dark brown, a complete bedroom set. She also has lots of souvenirs from places she visited on her trips, such as hats and clothes from Puerto Rico and Mexico. Her room has a lot of pictures of friends and family members, along with a few stuffed animals. Her clothes match her shoes, boots, sandals, and jewels. Her books are orderly. She has religious items including a silver rosary, a Bible, a few candles, the image of Virgen de Guadalupe, and a beautiful Crucifix next to her bed. All of her memories and significant items are with us forever. We recently gave away her clothes and other items after three years of her death.

She brought a lot of happiness through her facial expressions, big smile, good attitude, compassion, and warm personality. She was always ready to help others. She lived life to the fullest extent and accomplished many things. Our hearts and minds will forever be full of love for Nikalette. Our home is not the same. She is gone to heaven, and we thank God for those seventeen years of Nikalette. Now she is with us with Fotos, memories, and her spirit.

"I consider that the suffering of this present time
is as nothing compared with the glory to be
revealed for us by our Lord Jesus Christ."
- Romans 8:18

This Bible scripture provided us with some consolation. I know Nikalette is in heaven and she is our guardian angel—and that includes her classmates, friends, and family. Nikalette lived her life by assisting others thanks to her strong connection with Lord Jesus Christ; she is a model for all of us to follow.

As a registered nurse, I have learned how to deal with numerous crises and ongoing stress in a hospital setting, but nothing I learned during my career can compare to the true pain of what occurred within my own home. However, this situation did motivate me to do extensive research on epilepsy, and everything I've learned has increased my deep desire to guide others, while sharing my own experiences, through this book. I hope that my research and my own experience as a seasonal nurse can limit or decrease injuries and possible sudden deaths. The more knowledge we gain, the better care we can provide for our loved ones who suffer from epilepsy.

This true-life story illustrates our strong faith in God, which still, up to this day, is helping our family and friends cope with the death of Nikalette. All of us, up to this day, wonder what we could have done differently to save her life.

CHAPTER 2

Inspiration

What Nikalette Did to Inspire Others

Nikalette was a friendly person who provided a warm smile when she met new students, friends, and families. I remember the words she used to advise friends and classmates: "Do your best with any task or activity in life that you are given, but first develop a relationship with God for His help, as I have done. Keep in mind that any good, or not particularly good, action will affect our future." She emphasized to her brothers, sisters, friends, and classmates the need to develop a strong faith in and love for God and to have compassion for others. Strong faith would help them when they suffered disappointments in life. Nikalette faithfully prayed every morning and night. Before she went to school, we prayed together as part of our daily routine; her favorite prayers were the Lord's Prayer in the morning and the rosary in the evening. She attended Mass weekly and sought to bring along her brothers, sisters, and friends. She spoke to them about the importance of developing a spiritual life.

She was a child of God with all those spiritual gifts and made a significant impact on her family, classmates, friends, and her community. For her, everyone was a child of God. She wanted to include people from different backgrounds. She was unbiased and treated all people with respect, dignity, and love, especially those who were disabled, elderly or of different races, and of low social status. To her a person's educational level, religion, gender, or age did not matter. She had a good relationship with everyone such as children, adolescents, adults, and older adults.

No matter how difficult the situation was, she would help people. She asked us to help too. I recall one day she told me one of the new students in the school spoke mostly Arabic, with only limited knowledge of English. She was able to assist him and provided him with a tour of the school and included him in school activities so he would not feel out of place. She told me he was very appreciative.

One of my grandsons, Esteban, has autism. At times he can be challenging with his behavior. Nikalette always took care of him. She always wanted Esteban close to her so he would be supervised. She assisted him as needed, especially when we had family reunions or birthdays and holidays to celebrate. Esteban was extremely happy with Nikalette, and up to this day, he asks us for Nikalette.

She was able to turn negative situations into positive ones with her good character. As an example, two of her classmates did not get along at school. So Nikalette spoke first to one of them because they were assigned to do a project for science class as a team. Then she spoke to her other friend, Maria, and invited both of them to come to my house to work on the project. They all did well on the project and got outstanding grades. After we buried her, I became aware that she donated blood to people in need. She was always taking care of others before her own health needs. She was a warrior princess who accomplished more than the average person her age.

At times I wonder if she had an idea that she may not be with us for a long time, because she made a lot of repeated requests to me—for example, to make sure her siblings and classmates would continue with their faith in God, as community volunteers, and with their school responsibilities. It is very sad to see several of Nikalette's classmates, including her younger brother Sean, drop out of high school. Nikalette's determined mindset and energy were gifts from God, and it reflects through the following Scripture:

"They that hope in the Lord will renew their strength, they will soar on eagle's wings;
They will run and not grow weary,
walk and not grow faint."

- *Isaiah 40:31*

People noticed when she walked into a room. Nikalette would light it up with her inner and outer self. I do recall one time we went to a party and several people wanted a picture of Nikalette. They thought she was a Hollywood star because she dressed very elegantly, especially that day; she had on a beautiful blue summer dress, sunglasses, a nice scarf, and of course her enlightened personality. She stood out with her long brown hair and big hazel eyes.

Nikalette's Achievements Inspired Her Classmates

She encouraged others to do an excellent job, leading with her example. She persuaded others to do their best with love and a good attitude. Ever since Nikalette attended elementary school, she had excellent grades. She had a high-grade point average of 3.85 out of 4.0. She challenged herself by taking on more responsibilities. She sometimes felt like she needed more challenges and wanted to accomplish the maximum.

Nikalette was a cheerleader captain in preschool and first, second, and fifth grade and participated in several competitions that took place in suburbs close to Chicago such as Indiana, Yorkville, Oswego, and Aurora. She joined a dance team in preschool but stopped after second grade. Nikalette also participated in gymnastics and played flute and piano for a short period, until she was diagnosed with epilepsy. However, after entering high school, she did not continue with gymnastics or musical instruments so that she could continue with other sports and community volunteer work. She earned recognition in volleyball, soccer, and cross country. Her favorite sport was soccer; she was a defensive midfielder and played a very shorth period.

Starting in third grade, she was on seizure precaution and could not go on trips for sports or other activities. Although it was risky, Nikalette still enjoyed participating in those activities; she mentioned that it helped relieve her anxiety regarding being epileptic. Epilepsy did not stop Nikalette from enjoying school, sports, and music. She represented her school in many ways, and she still felt the need to do more.

On April 10, 2018, she was invited to the 2018 Distinguished Hall of Honor Assembly at Aurora West High School. She was in the second semester of her junior year. Due to Nikalette's strong GPA, she was asked to participate in this event. She was so happy to attend this assembly and felt very motivated to continue doing her best at school. Sadly this was only a month prior to Nikalette's departure to heaven. She did receive from God immeasurable grace to be happy and prosperous in her youth, which is why she succeeded with any task she took on. She was a young lady influencing others. Since she excelled in her studies, it was anticipated that she would graduate one semester early, in December 2018, with a high-grade point average in honor classes.

She had a talent for painting. She always designed posters for us to congratulate our friends on birthdays or graduation. She was a very initiative-taking girl. Students from her high school wrote letters and made two big posters describing Nikalette as "High spirited, sweet, athletic, productive, helpful, positive, humble, optimistic, curious, smart, determined, dedicated, honest, persistent, creative, grateful, excited, ambitious, inspiring, vibrant, well dressed, stylish, humorous, appreciative, cheerful, joyful, bright, active, thoughtful, big hearted, easy going and very spiritual." They all signed their names and included a beautiful picture of Nikalette in the center. On the day of Nikalette's school memorial service, the classmates gave us the posters. We were consoled by the songs of the school choir and all the one hundred people who attended this memorial on May 20, 2018, at 1 PM. The choir wore white and red to coordinate outfits. This service was very well done by her teachers and the staff from District 129 at Aurora West High School. Nikalette's family is extremely appreciative of this very impressive memorial service. All three schools that she attended also lowered the American flag in honor of Nikalette's life. That 2017–2018 high school yearbook had a special dedication to Nikalette. It had pictures of Nikalette, allowing students to remember my granddaughter forever. She helped everyone and brought a positive energy to the team. She really left a mark in her high school and on myself. She was funny, independent, gorgeous, respectful, charming, and determined. She will never be forgotten.

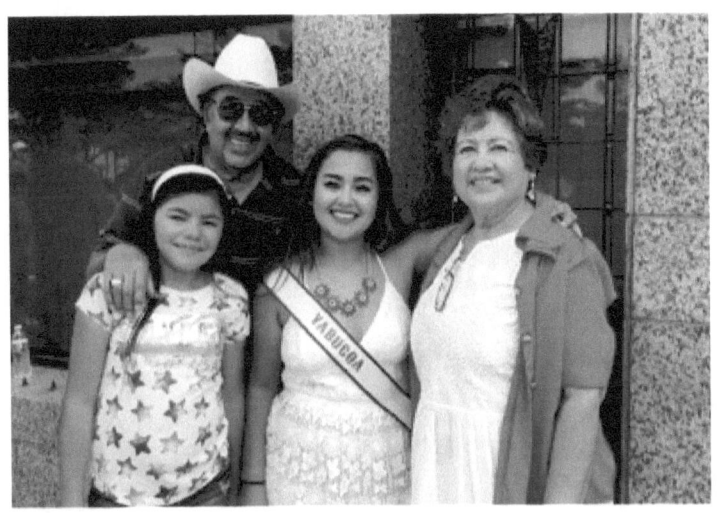

"Nikalette represents Yabucoa, Puerto Rico,
with Angelna, her younger sister,
and her grandparents."
July 2017.

CHAPTER 3

The Birth of the Warrior Princess

Nikalette was born on March 6, 2001, at Provena Mercy Hospital in Aurora, Illinois (a Catholic hospital which is now called Ascension Mercy Medical Center). Her mother, Sandra (Sandy) Simental Rangel, is Mexican American, while her father, Ramon Luis Rivera, was Puerto Rican. She was pleased with her heritage: bilingual and bicultural. She did school presentations for her Spanish class about being a Latina.

Nikalette's parents were thrilled and anxious while waiting for her to arrive. Sandy was admitted to the prenatal floor on March 5 around 7 PM. Both Ramon and I were with her at the time of admission. The doctor informed us that baby Nikalette would not come until the following day because the contractions were slow. The hospital policy allowed only one person to stay with the mother overnight, so Ramon stayed with Sandy. The doctor informed me that they would call me when the time came. Before I left for the night, we prayed together for a healthy outcome. I returned to the hospital very early the following day, on March 6, around 4 AM. I was surprised but relieved to find out that Nikalette had been born at 1:30 AM since I had not received a call from the hospital informing me that Nikalette was delivered. Sandy had a standard delivery with no complications. She also mentioned that the hospital was hectic during the night.

I was delighted that Ramon was there with Sandy throughout the night. He never left her side for one minute. I remember Ramon holding Nikalette in his arms while walking around the postpartum room. He was so happy and proud, looking into Nikalette's face. He seemed so relieved and satisfied that everything had gone well.

He said that Nikalette opened her eyes, looked at him, and smiled. Somehow, they had an immediate father and daughter bond, not knowing that he would only be in her life for less than a year. Ramon told me that day that he prayed his daughter would be just like me, that one day she would be close to God. He looked at me and said, "Since Sandy became pregnant, I wanted a girl." Ramon also told me he wanted his daughter to be a spiritual and loving girl like me. Still, I said to him that I also wanted her to be like him, with a strong faith in God, and to look like him, especially with hazel eyes, which she did have.

Ramon told us that he always loved Nikalette just as he loved all his other children. He already had two sons and two daughters and was an immensely proud father. He said that all his children would become close and love each other one day. We were all filled with joy when Nikalette smiled at us. She knew our love for her. Ramon told us multiple times, "I always will love Nikalette as I love the rest of my kids."

Nikalette admired and deeply loved both her father's and mother's families. She felt incredibly proud of them and had an excellent relationship with them. Her oldest stepsister from her father's family, Janessa, is in the nursing profession in Tampa, Florida, and has two beautiful daughters. Nikalette loved her two adorable nieces and became remarkably attached to them when she visited her family in Florida. She also had two stepbrothers, Junito and Cesar, and a stepsister, Raquel. On her mother's side, Nikalette has a stepbrother, Sam Anthony, who studies accounting and health care administration. Her siblings Sean and Angelina are younger and attend high school. All of them were doing well, but Sean decided to drop out of West Aurora High School four weeks before graduation in May 2022 to get a job and live with his girlfriend at the age of eighteen.

Ever since her birth, Nikalette was always a healthy and happy child. She always had a positive expression on her beautiful face and rarely cried. When Nikalette was only ten months old, she lost her father due to septicemia. He had a small abrasion on his leg was told by my daughter Sandy y my nephew a medical student to see a doctor immediately but he refused. That infection in two days got worse. Ramon went to the hospital on the third day and died in the emergency room. I do remember that day. We had to inform Nikalette that her father had gone away for a trip. She cried and cried the whole day, and nothing would comfort her. It was as if she knew that her father would no longer be in her life; it was heartbreaking. My husband immediately tried to provide a father's love to her. Nikalette saw her grandfather as her father. Nikalette used to visit the gravesite of her father Ramon at the cemetery in Aurora, especially on Father's Day or around Christmas, and would bring flowers. Nikalette once told me, "I wish my father Ramon was alive so he could see I am doing well, and he would feel proud of his Puerto Rican daughter." I replied, "Your father's spirit is with you." Nikalette also used to tell me, "I am doing all this work to please God, and I want my father who is in heaven and the rest of my family to be proud of me." She was highly active and happy despite the loss of her father. She always had her father Ramon in her mind. She always wanted to know more about him. She became close to all people from Puerto Rico and got angry when people told her she was not really Puerto Rican, because she was so proud of her heritage. Now she is with her father Ramon, whom she loves, forever.

Ramon and Sandy met after they were finalizing their respective divorces from their first marriages. They started dating and moved to Clearwater, Florida, without getting married, but then a few months later they returned to Aurora. It appears to me that they did not get along, and they were separated when Nikalette was a newborn; however, Ramon took care of Nikalette until his death when Nikalette was only 10 months. He was a good father to all his children.

Ever since she was a year old, Nikalette loved to listen to Christian music, especially "Amazing Grace" and "Ave Maria." In my home, we play a lot of Christian music. I remember one time when she was about three years old, we were in my car, and I had nonreligious music turned on. She asked me to change the radio because she wanted something different. Because she was young, though, it was hard for me to understand what she wanted exactly. I kept turning on the radio, but she would cry and say "no . . . no" until I finally played "Ave Maria." It was only then that she stopped crying. She was pleased and calm, so we played it repeatedly for her to enjoy.

Nikalette walked and talked before she was a year old. She was in the daycare center starting at seven months old, and she learned to speak both English and Spanish. At home, we speak Spanish most of the time. At eighteen months, her teacher told Sandy that they would transition Nikalette into the older children's class. Her teacher felt that Nikalette needed more of a challenge, and she adapted well. She quickly learned the alphabet, colors, and numbers and played well with the new group of older children. Nikalette took on more tasks including helping other children and comforting them.

Nikalette went to the KinderCare Learning Center in Aurora for all her preschool years. There she met a sweet, special girl named Briana, who was the same age as her. They were remarkably close childhood friends. They would share toys and play together all the time. Nikalette's favorite toys were baby dolls. They also shared parties and other children's activities outside the Kinder-Care. They loved each other so much that they never got tired of playing together. Briana developed epilepsy early, and Nikalette was highly concerned about her friend's health. We visited Briana at her home when she did not go to the daycare center—not knowing that Nikalette would also be impacted with epilepsy years later.

Once Nikalette was diagnosed with epilepsy, she became closer to Briana and her family. The girls' friendship grew, and we were all there to help support each other through everything. Nikalette and Briana were friends up to the day Nikalette died. Briana and her mother attended the funeral service on May 16, 2018, and both of them attended Nikalette's memorial service at Aurora West High School on May 20, 2016. Briana and her mother were also present at the Puerto Rico parade on

July 29, 2018, one section of this celebration was to honor Nikalette's life.

Nikalette was enthusiastic and extremely popular in her school. She touched so many people with her positive qualities. She was even a rowdy football supporter. She was loud and spirited at her high school games, always with a smile in her warm personality to encourage students to reach their goals in everything from academics to sports.

She was determined to succeed. If she was unsure about a school assignment, she would consult me. In addition, she spent prolonged hours in the library. She would read, research, and analyze articles for her school assignments and papers. Her research papers had to be perfect. She attended extra classes if more support was needed. Overall she was a dedicated student and was preparing for her career one day.

I recall that there was a time when she had to do a project regarding the planets of the solar system and the phases of meteors. It had to explain how the meteors burn up before hitting the earth, causing no damage to our environment. She was in seventh grade at the time. The science project was well done. She put many hours and effort into designing this project that contained so many details, and she presented it in front of her classmates. Her teacher liked it so much that she asked Nikalette if she would like to donate it to the class for the rest of the students to look at and learn from. Her project served as didactic material, a tool for learning. Of course, Nikalette agreed and was so happy about it. When she came home and informed me, she said she wanted to make it easier for the other students to enjoy learning. She wanted to convey that acquiring new knowledge can be fun.

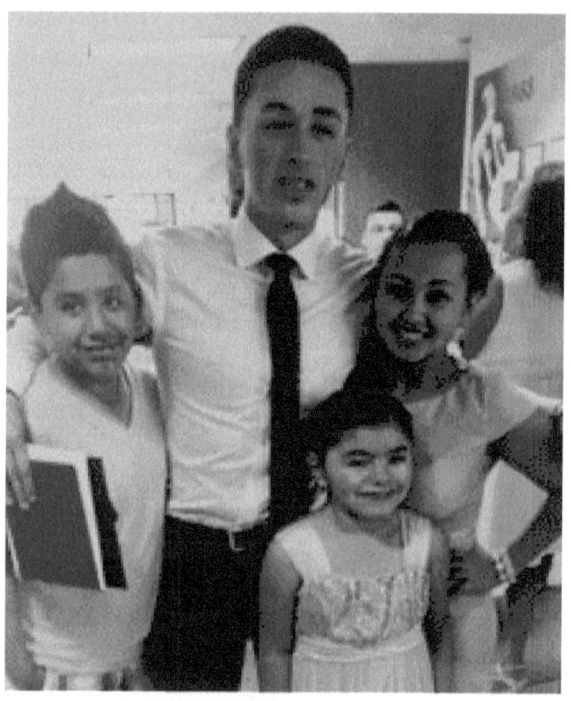

From left to right Sean, Sam, Nikalette, and Angelina, June 2016.
Sam high school Graduation.

CHAPTER 4

Amazing Life

Growing Up with Her Mother, Siblings, and Grandparents

The rich memories of Nikalette's amazing life are in my mind every second, every minute, and every hour and forever will be with me. Her oldest brother, Sam Anthony, was born December 27, 1996. Nikalette was born March 6, 2001. Sean Michael was born October 28, 2004, and Angelina was born July 31, 2006.

Nikalette's father Ramon had two sons and two daughters from a previous marriage; most of this lovely family is in Tampa, Florida, though one sister of the sisters is in Plano, Illinois.

When my husband and I retired, we had the opportunity to move to another state or country for our golden years. Yet we decided to stay here in Illinois to be close to Nikalette, our other grandchildren, family, long-term friends, and our church group. We thank God that we are healthy and are able to serve others.

My daughter Sandy has four children and assisted to raise Jordan; she had been a single parent for the past thirteen years, all of them were living in our home with exception of Jordan he went to Texas with his father George Ochoa he was the second husband of Sandy. My husband and I assisted my daughter Sandy in raising her children; they learned religion, morals, and family values with discipline, love, and respect for others. We attended church activities and did community volunteer work. On weekends we spent time at church, with God as the first priority, but also made time for family, friends, eating out, and working out at the gym.

I also took Nikalette to school when I was not working. At times we struggled since we all worked full time. Sandy had two jobs in critical care and on the medical-surgical floor. I was the assistant unit director for the medical surgical rehabilitation nursing units at Rush University Medical Center in Chicago. Later I was promoted to staff educator for the medical-surgical rehabilitation nursing units, and I did my best. We all worked different hours to be available to take care of the family, and we provided the care and a safe environment for my daughter's kids.

Nikalette and I shopped together for groceries, sports items, dresses, and school supplies. We went to the store to find a dress for the formal party we had to celebrate my husband's and my fiftieth wedding anniversary. I went to the women's section, and Nikalette went to the juniors' section. We met in the women's fitting area and were surprised that we chose the same dress in the same color and style, except mine was a few sizes bigger. We started laughing and joking around. She said, "We have similar interests in dresses." When we tried the dresses on, she looked beautiful hers, though unfortunately my dress did not fit me. I bought her a beautiful dress, and she wore it for my anniversary.

Occasionally, we went to the Olive Garden for pasta and salads. We also enjoyed Puerto Rican criollo food, such as pastel, rellenos de papa (stuffed potatoes), pernil (ham), arroz con habichuelas (rice with beans), and tostones (plantain chips). Mexican food was also delicious, and we loved dishes such as tamales, mole, and tacos (traditionally made with small hand-sized corn or wheat tortillas, topped with chicken and vegetables), and chicken wings as well. We visited restaurants in Aurora and Chicago, her favorite places. Usually, we had a good time even though there were stressful days, like after a seizure when she could not eat but still wanted to join us. Our mealtimes together would sometimes be interrupted when she received a phone call from a friend who needed help with schoolwork or who just wanted to talk to us. An anecdote that always made us laugh was from when she was seven years old and she jumped off a swing and landed right on her face. She always remembered that fall because she got a small bruise on one of her cheeks.

One of her hobbies was reading all kinds of books, but the one she enjoyed the most was *The Fault in Our Stars* by John Green. Her favorite songs were by One Direction, Drake, and Taylor Swift.

In addition to reading, Nikalette also enjoyed making others happy. There was a ceremony held when she finished at Jefferson Middle School in Aurora. All the students had a pretty yellow rose, and their teacher and school principal asked the students to give the rose to the person they admired as a good role model to continue education. I was stunned and honored when she brought the rose to me; she told me how much she loved me and that she would be just like me in their future. We hugged each other with teary eyes.

I enjoyed all those hours that we did spend together with Nikalette. She was charming. She did ask me questions regarding my nursing studies and my relationship with my husband and my friends. One time I brought her to the Greek Islands restaurant on Halsted Street in Chicago where I met several nurses from Rush hospital for dinner. She had a nice time and was mature and well-behaved. She brought so much joy into our lives through her easy-going nature, intelligence, and kindness. I miss her a lot.

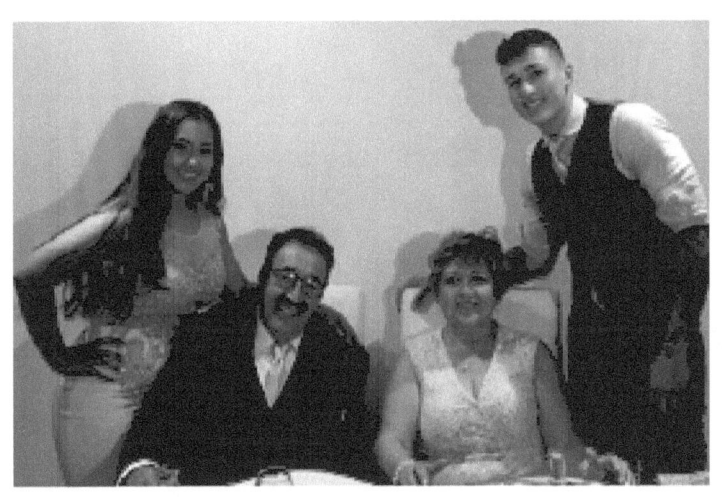

*"Celebration of our fiftieth anniversary with
Nikalette, Juan, Lilia, and Sam Anthony, her older brother in
Mexico."*

2017

CHAPTER 5

Nocturnal Seizures, Home Interventions, and a Service Dog

Interventions for Seizures and Nikalette's Fear of Bullying

In April 2009, Nikalette had an incredibly stressful day. Her stepfather and her mother were arguing in front of her at home, which made her terribly upset and highly nervous. Though she said nothing that evening, she had been quiet and worried about everything that happened that day. When she went to sleep that night, she experienced a grand mal seizure for the first time. She was nine years old and at the time she was attending Freeman Elementary School. She was a healthy person, never sick until that time. Sandy took her to the doctor the next day, and she was given an anticonvulsant. Nikalette was hospitalized for one week at the Children's Hospital in Park Ridge. Nikalette learned that her diagnosis of epilepsy was a chronic disease and that she would experience seizure episodes during the night. She regularly saw her neurologist and had a blood test and an electroencephalogram (EEG) every month. At times, the lab procedures were completed at Rush Copley in Aurora as well.

She was overly concerned and afraid to tell people about her seizures, especially her classmates or new friends. She was worried that she would face bullying or discrimination. We agreed to keep her diagnosis confidential, but later in life she gained confidence. She would say, "Now that I am epileptic, I have more faith in God. He wants me to be His instrument to guide others with love and understanding to be very serious about life. One day I will treat epileptic people just like me." Although Nikalette was experiencing this new medical challenge, she was still thinking of how to support others.

I am asking readers now to please stop any inappropriate behavior toward or intimidation of anyone with an illness or disability. Making fun of them is not acceptable. One cannot control the cause of abnormal walking, talking, muscle twitching, or being in a wheelchair. Some may have special needs due to physical impairments. As a nurse, I know they are already suffering from chronic illness, disability, or other problems. If their symptoms rub you the wrong way, please ignore them or look away. With respect, I am asking you to end all mistreatment, discrimination, or bullying of people for the way they are. Nikalette was very fearful of suffering intimidation due to her epilepsy. Remember, God loves all of us, and we are all precious in our Lord's eyes. We do not need to put anyone down for us to feel better. Praying is extremely helpful. We need to be grateful for our health, especially when we have sadness and hardship during a global pandemic. God walks with us all the time.

Nikalette's health condition was risky, so she was not allowed to go over to her friends' houses. Instead, Nikalette invited classmates and friends into our house. Some friends needed a ride home, so we were happy to do them the favor, while others would spend the night with their parents' permission. Several girls even stayed over for a couple of nights; a few of these include Monica, Charisma, Jasmin, Samantha, and Alexa. They would do homework and school projects, and of course other teenage activities like doing their hair, talking, and watching TV. They had a fun time. I always supervised them, and if they had questions regarding anything, I helped them. Sometimes I researched to find the correct answer. It was fun to be around young teenagers.

Diagnosis

When Nikalette was first diagnosed, her medications often had to be adjusted, so doctors' visits were more frequent than when she got older. She took 1,000 mg Levetiracetam in the morning and 1,500 mg at bedtime and clonazepam while on her menstrual cycle. Her doctor adjusted her meds following her blood tests and her seizures. Nikalette luckily responded well to her medications.

She had a daily routine. We made sure she took her medication prior to school and before going to bed. She had three healthy meals. After she completed her homework, she went to the gym to exercise for one hour and then showered. It was most important for her to have a good night's sleep, especially after a stressful day. She loved to study and never got tired of it. I even had to tell her to stop reading and go to sleep because I was concerned about sleep deprivation. Overwhelming days were one of the triggers for her seizures.

A Service Dog for Nikalette

We also had a service dog named Bruno in our home for several years. For those of you who do not know, a service dog is trained to assist people with disabilities and is protected by the American Disability Act (ADA) laws here in the United States. Assistance animals' or service dogs' functions and registration, policies, and procedures depend on each country. Bruno was a beautiful brown Pitbull, a unique and lovely dog. If you saw his angry face, you would want to run away from him. But if he knew you, he was friendly and particularly good at alerting us to any danger. Bruno was a good dog. He would bark and bark to protect any family member, especially Nikalette. Bruno stayed in Nikalette's room during the night and would always warn us when she had a seizure. He became part of our family, and we slept better when he was around. We felt safe with him because he would alert us immediately if Nikalette had a seizure. He would run to either Sandy's room or my room and then direct us to Nikalette. He would not stop barking until Nikalette was OK. Unfortunately, Bruno died before Nikalette.

Once Bruno was no longer around, we used a noise monitor. The microphone was attached to Nikalette's bed while the speaker was in my bedroom. Her bedroom door was always open and a phone was next to her bed. I thank God that I was able to monitor her every night. Many nights, if I heard a noise through the noise monitor, I would immediately run into her room to assess Nikalette for seizures. Then she would wake up and ask me what I was doing in her room. She was uncomfortable and anxious, and I told her to go to sleep and not to worry. My daughter Sandy and I trained family members, friends, and even classmates on seizure precautions. We wanted to prevent Nikalette from sustaining any injury. One family member would stay in Nikalette's room during the night to supervise and assist Nikalette if needed.

Whichever family member stayed with Nikalette during the night knew that if she had any seizure activity, they were responsible for turning her onto her side to drain her mouth secretions, so that she would not drown or aspirate. When Nikalette had a grand mal seizure, she would sometimes have a loud cry prior to the seizure. Then the seizure activity occurred. Other times there were no signs or symptoms to let us know about an upcoming seizure episode. Her extremities got stiff, then started twitching, especially the right side. She would have difficulty breathing, which would lead to her going unconscious. When those seizures happened, she was never incontinent or had any bowel and bladder accidents, but she did go into convulsions. It was excruciating to see her suffering. She then experienced postictal nausea, vomiting, headache, fatigue, or disorientation before falling into a deep sleep. However, the next morning she was ready to start her day with a lot of energy and joy. We would place pillows around her bed to maintain a safe environment in case she would fall out. Nikalette's seizures lasted anywhere from fifty seconds to three minutes. A couple times, we had to call 911, and the paramedics would take Nikalette by ambulance to the emergency room if she had a prolonged seizure or if she turned blue or became stiff. The ambulance took her to the nearby hospital for an emergency visit, but luckily, she was usually discharged the same day, only needing a follow-up appointment with her neurologist.

CHAPTER 6

Leader for West Aurora High School

Most of the time, Nikalette functioned as a leader at school. Although an honor student, she still was humble and remarkably close to God. She became a Link Leader, setting an example by doing her best academically. A Link Leader required the upper-level students to welcome and help the first- and second-year students at West Aurora High School. The leaders were academic tutors for those who needed support with research projects and other assignments, and they also encouraged the underclassmen to participate in sports or in other productive activities. She directed these younger students to the proper counselors and teachers if they needed emotional support.

Her classmates called Nikalette a compassionate and energetic leader. Because of these many groups, my house was always filled with students invited by Nikalette.

"Success is not just about what you accomplish in your life, but success is what you inspire others to do" was Nikalette's favorite quote, the one she used when working as a leader with her classmates, friends, and siblings. When encountering difficult problems, she did not give up but instead stayed focused and did her research. It was inspirational to see Nikalette's strong passion to assist others in their education.

Nikalette was not only a leader at school, but also with her family, especially with her siblings and cousins. She was a highly organized person and offered to help the family get organized. For example, she would ask what everybody would like to do for Thanksgiving, Christmas, New Year's, Easter, or birthday parties. Then she would write out the responsibilities for these parties, making lists of all the activities and preparation required for the meals and would assign tasks to different members of the family. She guided and assisted others in numerous activities, and after doing her assignments, she would follow up with a call or a text message to make sure that no one forgot anything. So our celebrations were always fun and went smoothly.

Nikalette was well known, loved, and respected by her classmates and our Aurora community. She was a light for other students, a mature soul who motivated them through her example of spirituality and discipline. She constantly encouraged others not to let anything interfere with their educational and professional goals and to accomplish the maximum they could. She told them, "I am here to help you with anything."

Since she wanted to go to medical school, Nikalette participated as a member of Health Occupations Students of America (HOSA) for future health professionals at her high school. That was one of her favorite classes. She loved, admired, and respected her teachers, Mrs. Sheila McQuade, her HOSA English teacher; Miss Smith, her chemistry teacher; her Spanish teacher; and many others. She talked to me about them and consulted me on any science or disease-related topics. She also respected her coaches and advisors at her high school. Nikalette always talked to me about her interaction with her teachers, exhibiting respect for them and admiration for her outstanding learning experiences, school activities, and friends. She was always studying and getting prepared for any test, and it did not matter how much energy it took. She would roll up her sleeves and get to work.

In February 2018, Nikalette visited three universities in Chicago. She ultimately planned to attend her first two years at Waubonsee Community College in Sugar Grove, Illinois, then finish the final two years at Aurora University where she would earn her bachelor's in science and biology. She even earned two scholarships from Aurora University. She had actually already taken a few classes at Waubonsee Community College and Aurora University, so she was familiar with both places. Then she planned to transfer to Loyola University in Chicago, Illinois, for medical school. She was highly impressed by the Loyola University tour guide. She told me that Loyola University was highly organized and very professional, and she was happy that the campus was so close to Lake Michigan. It met all her expectations. Nikalette said, "They have a church on campus, Grandma, and I love it." Since she was very spiritual, she felt she needed it to be close to God. She wanted to attend Mass regularly, since she always attended church in Aurora, Naperville, or Batavia.

She had a plan for her future and was determined to accomplish it. She wrote two letters to me and told me when to open them. She wanted me to open the first one when she completed her university degree and the second letter when she finished medical school. I still have those letters and others notes that she wrote to me to let me know how appreciative she was of us. One of the reasons she wanted to go to school close to home was her epilepsy.

I think her close relationship with God, the fact that she did not have her father in her life and being impacted with epilepsy all definitely helped her to grow up faster. She did become closer to God for spiritual support at an early age. Then she focused on guiding others in the appropriate direction.

Community Involvement

Our family was engaged in community service, and we demonstrated to Nikalette the importance of helping others in need. Our philosophy is that, when we volunteer, our lives truly have value, purpose, and meaning. If we are blessed, we must be a blessing to others. Happiness and satisfaction are achieved when we connect ourselves to our creator, our heavenly Father, Jesus Christ.

We have multiple professionals in our family, such as teachers, engineers, professors, and doctors, who served as role models to Nikalette. Her uncles and aunts also help people in the community. Most of them work in hospitals and schools. I am a recently retired registered nurse but still volunteer at church, as a home health nurse, and at hospitals within the community.

Nikalette volunteered at Hesed House, a homeless shelter in Aurora, for five years, once a month on Saturdays. People still miss her. She helped in the kitchen preparing fruits and vegetables and served food to the people in the shelter. Once everyone was done eating, she would help clean the kitchen and the tables; her mother Sandy also volunteered at the shelter and was able to assist and supervise Nikalette as needed.

While she was running for the Miss Puerto Rico pageant, she had monthly meetings and other responsibilities in the town of Aurora, for example, feeding the poor and sick people or occasionally visiting patients at the nursing homes. She also participated in cultural community events to represent Aurora's Puerto Rican and Latinx communities.

Nikalette also participated in the community Easter celebration in our Prestbury subdivision in Sugar Grove. Easter is a yearly Christian event that celebrates the resurrection of Jesus Christ which occurred three days after His crucifixion. In April 2016, Nikalette helped our community with the Easter decorations and enjoyed coloring eggs before the event. She also helped by supervising and assisting anywhere from fifty to eighty children of all different ages on Easter Day.

Nikalette always loved working with children. She told me that she wanted to take her little cousin Victoria, who was just one year old in 2016, for the next Easter celebration in 2017. Nikalette was already close to Victoria, my youngest granddaughter. However, even though she was walking by that year, Victoria did not attend the Easter celebration in 2017 because she was sick that day.

Nikalette told other students and her friends to develop a deep faith in God and to be strong and positive even when faced with disappointing experiences. She believed in having the discipline to reach her goals and encouraged this in others as well. She was always happy and lived the way she wanted to live. She was also very responsible and rarely missed school, church, or sports activities unless she had doctor's appointments. A few times she was grounded at home if she would not listen, or if she wanted to go out with her friends but not return home until 11 PM even though she needed to be in bed by 10 PM. Other times she did raise her voice to us, but then we removed her phone privileges for a day or two (depending on the situation). Although she would be upset for an hour or so, she always apologized to us. She was after all just an adolescent girl who wanted to do what her friends were doing, but she knew the importance of getting her sleep to prevent seizures.

Occasionally Nikalette would babysit for children in our neighborhood, and her classmates and friends would often stop by our home if they needed a safe person to talk to for advice or a prayer. A month before Nikalette's death, she told me that one of her friends had committed suicide. She was heartbroken and told me we needed to do more for her friends and classmates to stop suicidal ideation. I know she was grieving. But she never complained of being tired.

CHAPTER 8

Nikalette's Sacraments

Nikalette grew in her faith through her sacraments. Her Baptism, First Communion, and Confirmation were all celebrated at Saint Rita of Cascia Catholic Church. Her baptism was on August 19, 2001, with her godparents (padrinos), Al Medernach and Connie Rangel. Her First Communion was on May 20, 2009, and my husband and I were her godparents. Then her Confirmation was on October 21, 2017, and her godmother (madrina) was Lilly Alvarez, her aunt. The religious ceremony was administered by Bishop David J. Malloy.

The church was packed as approximately two hundred students received the sacrament of Confirmation in a beautiful ceremony. We felt the Holy Spirit was with us, seeing all the young students following faith and God. Although it took two years of Confirmation classes and Bible studies in preparation to receive this sacrament, Nikalette was happy. She had perfect attendance for her First Communion, Confirmation, and Bible classes. She was very dedicated, determined, and diligent in doing every task assigned to her. She wrote a research paper for her Bible class on the Gospel of St. Luke because he was a doctor. Relatives and friends attended her Confirmation celebration, took pictures, and celebrated in a nice restaurant for dinner. She read her confirmation certificate to us as follows: "Nikalette was sealed with the gift of the Holy Spirit and was confirmed in faith in the name of the Father, Son, and the Holy Spirit." Nikalette continued reading what was read to her at church: "Come, Holy Spirit, fill the hearts of the faithful and kindle in them the fire of your love."

Nikalette did ask me many times to make sure that her younger brother Sean and her younger sister Angelina would complete their confirmation program; she wanted them to be as close to our Lord Jesus Christ as she was. It's as if she knew she would not be here for them. Several times I promised her that I would be responsible for making sure her younger siblings attended their Religious Education classes as she had done. My promise is completed now that they celebrated their Confirmation on November 21, 2020, at St. Rita Church.

Nikalette also attended Calvary Temple, a beautiful church in Naperville, Illinois. She was hungry to learn more about Jesus Christ. She said, "Grandma, I feel the presence of God in my life even in my low times. I feel the presence of the Holy Spirit, especially when I'm praying."

Nikalette even attended a third church, Holy Cross in Batavia, Illinois, on Wednesdays for the Eucharistic Adoration, when Our Lord is truly present to us, even though we don't see Him. We can feel His presence. Nikalette attended church regularly; she was an excellent Catholic Christian girl. Nikalette was surrounded by a caring Catholic Christian family and developed her knowledge, values, and morals.

After her death, I regretted that I had not sent her to a Catholic school for her education, as she always wanted and had asked me to do multiple times. Although she enjoyed and loved her excellent teachers and classmates in her public schools, she missed the religion context and Bible classes. She wanted to be closer to God and grow deeper in her faith in Jesus Christ. She placed Him first. One of her favorite scriptures from the Holy Bible was Philippians 4:13. It was all over her room, inside her books, and in her prayers: "I have the strength for everything through him who empowers me."

My husband and I have been married for more than fifty years, and we do not want our adult children to have the burden of making decisions at the last minute. So on May 20, 2017, we bought two plots in a cemetery close to our house in Sugar Grove. Since we are up in age and have already lost several family members younger than us, we decided to prepare for heaven. The Lord can call us at any time. Nikalette caught me looking at the cemetery map when she arrived home from school one day, and she was in shock. She asked me what I was doing. I responded, "We just bought two plots for my husband and me, so when the Lord calls us to be with him, we will be ready. Since we have been together for a long time, we want to be buried at the same place."

Nikalette responded, "No, please, no. I do not want to lose any of you, and you are like my parents. I need both of you, and I love you very much. I want you to be at my graduation from high school, college, and medical school, and when I get married. Both of you are healthy. You will be with me for a long time. Please, we don't think about dying." Then she kissed me and left the room, not knowing that the next year, in the same month, she would be buried in one of those plots; what irony is this life? Those plots were supposed to be for my husband and me, but the funeral home the manager told me that we could still be together in the same plot. After we die, one of us will be cremated while the other will be buried. We would be placed together next to our warrior princess, Nikalette, since we assisted my daughter in raising her. We are very close to Nikalette, and we will ever be.

Several days after Nikalette died, Sandy, her mother, was crying uncontrollably and would not stop. We did not know how to console her. Suddenly we heard Nikalette's phone ringing and ringing. Finally Sandy answered it. It was an incredible Holy Bible reading for that day, of Philippians 4:10: "I rejoice greatly in the Lord that now at last you revived your concern for me."

We did not realize until that day that Nikalette had registered on her phone for a daily Bible reading. Still, we knew about her strong faith in our Creator of the universe, our Lord Jesus Christ. Her faith in God was rock solid, nurtured by youth ministry programs, sacraments, and her spiritual family. So the verse consoled all of us. We knew that those daily Bible readings were helpful to my granddaughter, and now it was helpful to all of us as well. Her faith was the reason that she achieved multiple tasks that she endeavored.

Nikalette always prayed, asking God to cure her epilepsy. God did listen to her and took care of her seizures, but He also took her to be with Him. I am sure she is in heaven with Jesus Christ, living an eternal life with God, no longer suffering from seizures. Nikalette had complete trust in our Heavenly Father and Jesus Christ our Lord. Our family strongly believes in our Lord Jesus Christ, and I would not want to be in this world without my deep faith in God.

Every opportunity Nikalette had; she would pray. She mentioned to me several times that she felt the presence of God with her prayers. I told her to continue praying to enhance her faith. When my husband and I used to pray the rosary as a family, she would hear us and quietly sit next to us. She would begin praying the rosary in Spanish, even without our asking her to join us. She was the only grandchild who would pray the rosary in Spanish.

Nikalette also was happy to help me with any volunteer jobs for my church, and I always made the time to be with her. She used to tell me, "You are a registered nurse; my mom is a Certified Respiratory Therapist. Both of you need to teach me how to take care of patients because I will be a doctor of neurology." If I had a sick patient, she said, "please teach me so I can learn to take care of patients, grandma". At times I did talk to her about my experience as a nurse, and she was fascinated. I knew she had the compassion heart and the intelligence to be working in the hospital setting in the future. As you can see, the sacraments, attending church regularly, and participating in our community enhanced our faith in God. Those are the tools to live the kind of healthy and happy life that Nikalette lived.

CHAPTER 9

Canada and Mexico

I am thrilled that we took vacations with Nikalette, sometimes with the whole family and other times just with Nikalette and myself. We planned vacations together. She always brought several ideas, such as museums and speedboat trips, for tours and places to visit and assisted us in making flight reservations. She enjoyed traveling and enjoyed learning about different cultures. She was ready to go anywhere with the family. For our vacation trips, we visited places including Texas, Tennessee, New York, Tampa, and Florida; Canada; Veracruz, Torreón, Coahuila, and Durango, Mexico; and Puerto Rico. We traveled to the beach in Mazatlán and Veracruz, Mexico, just the two of us. I enjoyed those vacations so much.

Our trip to Toronto, Canada, was a fabulous experience. We visited Ontario and Niagara Falls in the summer of 2013. We rented an SUV for ten people: four grandchildren (Nikalette and her oldest brother Sam Anthony, plus two cousins, Khristian and Alex) and six adults (my son Juan Jr, his wife Veronica, two aunts—Socorro and Cristy—from Texas, and my husband and me). We drove from Chicago to Detroit, Michigan, then crossed the border to Canada. We spent six days vacationing in Canada.

We went to see fascinating places. We visited stores, several parks, and famous museums throughout Ontario and went sightseeing in Toronto. We visited Casa Loma, a Gothic Revival-style mansion and garden in midtown Toronto. Constructed between 1911 and 1914, it is now a historic house museum and landmark. We also visited Niagara Falls; with its magnificent view, Nikalette and I wanted to stay there for hours and hours. It was so fascinating in this beautiful place. We stayed at the Courtyard Marriott in Niagara Falls, Ontario.

Canada is a beautiful country with friendly people who did everything to accommodate our needs. Nikalette and all the rest of our family had a genuinely lovely trip. This vacation was an outstanding experience.

Mexico Trip with Nikalette

Nikalette and I also traveled to Mexico City for my nephew's graduation. We flew from Chicago O'Hare to Mexico D.F. in less than four hours. My nephew, Ernesto Jasiel Ibarra Rangel, graduated as a Mechatronic Engineer along with a multidisciplinary electrical and mechanic system branch. He had the highest-grade point average in his class. He speaks five languages, as he attended Universities in Poland and Germany for engineering. Nikalette asked him many questions about learning other languages in Europe. She was so impressed with him and told him that she would travel to Europe to learn other languages one day.

We attended his graduation on December 10, 2016, but first, we went to Mass at Our Lady of Rosary church at 7 PM. It is a tradition in Mexico to thank God for all the new graduating engineers. After the Mass, we went to a café opposite the Mural Salon between Acapulco, Guadalajara, and Durango Streets.

The graduation party was held in a beautiful place in Mexico D.F. The graduation ceremony was very well organized, and everything was done elegantly. Approximately one thousand people attended—two hundred graduates plus all the family members. The inside of the building was filled with paintings of famous artists from Israel. The organizers led us to our tables. Our dinner was delicious, and they had live music. Everyone dressed very elegantly, which was appropriate for this beautiful place. They also had an excellent orchestra. When it was over, we went back to the motel around 11:30 PM, as Nikalette needed to get her sleep. My nephew Jasiel informed us that the party did not end until 6 AM the next day when they served breakfast for all the new graduates and a mariachi band played.

Nikalette was curious and eager to learn about any place that she visited. She read about Mexico, the country, and its population, and she shared that information with the family group during dinner. She mentioned that Mexico, the country, has approximately more than 130 million people and its three biggest cities are Guadalajara, Jalisco; Monterrey, Nuevo León; and Mexico City (Distrito Federal). The City of Mexico Distrito Federal has a population of more than 20 million.

We stayed at the Zocalo motel in the center of Mexico City, close to the Basilica of Our Lady of Guadalupe. It is a famous church with multiple tourists and visitors from all over the world, especially in December. It is a very spiritual, sacred, and safe place to visit. It is well known around the world for daily miracles. More than twenty million people visit the Basilica every year; nine million come around December 12, to pray, receive blessings from our Virgen of Guadalupe, and see this holy place.

Nikalette wanted to know the entire story regarding the cathedral's history. She read books and learned why many people visited Mexico City in December. She was fascinated with everything. Spain ruled the land of Mexico for more than three hundred years until early 1800. The Indigenous people of Mexico were subjugated to the point that human sacrifice was practiced for religious beliefs. There was also suffering due to poverty and discrimination.

Our Mother of God appeared in the morning of December 9, 1531, to Juan Diego, a poor Aztec Indian. Three times he saw the apparition of Virgen, who was pregnant. She asked him to talk to the Bishop of Mexico City and tell them to build a church on the Tepeyac Hill of Mexico City. Juan Diego was very insecure, nervous, and unsure about doing this. Despite his misgivings, he went to the church and did what our Mother of God requested. No one believed him, so they asked him to bring proof. When he saw the Mother of God for the second time, he asked her to give him something to show to the bishop regarding her request. The Mother of God sent him miraculous flowers in his cloak to tell the bishop to build the church for the people to receive Her Son and Her loving spiritual care. On December 12, 1531, Juan Diego opened his cloak in front of the bishop. An image of the Mother of God was revealed and remains intact without any deterioration. The church was built immediately, and eight million people became Christians. The church increased the protection of the Indigenous, poor people and brought an end to the practice of human sacrifice. Juan Pablo II, our Polish Pope, visited this Cathedral in Mexico City several times and canonized Juan Diego as a saint in 2007.

Our visit to Mexico City was an excellent opportunity to see this church daily for Mass or to pray the rosary. Nikalette's father was devoted to Our Lady of Guadalupe, which was one of the reasons that Nikalette wanted to know the history. Her gravesite now has an image of the Virgin of Guadalupe.

CHAPTER 10

Celebration of Nikalette's Quinceañera in 2016

Nikalette had a very elegant quinceañera; this celebration is only for girls when they turn fifteen, a bit like a wedding party. It is a tradition in the Spanish culture that begins with a Mass to give thanks to God for everything she has in her life. Her party was at the Courtyard Banquets, in Warrenville, Illinois, and was attended by 175 people. It was held on July 29, 2016, about three months after her actual fifteenth birthday, to give time for many family members to travel from other cities and countries. There was a dinner and dance party, very well organized and elegant. Nikalette danced with fourteen of her childhood friends and classmates, seven girls and seven boys (damas y chambelanes). Everyone was dressed in white, and her dress was a beautiful long, pink ball gown. She had a special dance with her Uncle Pucho, who represented her father. She also danced with my husband, a tradition in the Spanish culture, as she was close to him. Finally, she danced with her mother, Sandy. They both looked beautiful, dancing together in their dresses of the same color. Nikalette changed to a shorter dress for some of her other Puerto Rican dance performances. Her fourteen friends wore white shorts and teal-colored T-shirts with their names on them. Linda White was the excellent dance teacher who choreographed their dances.

Nikalette had a cake from Orland Park Bakery; they are famous for their delicious cakes. Everyone got a chance to take professional pictures with her, and a lot of photos were taken both at church and at the banquet. The party was beautiful. Nikalette was happy and loved by all those who came in contact with her.

Nikalette was also very thankful that her special day was not canceled due to the tragic events of her oldest brother, Sam Anthony, which occurred weeks before.

My grandson is 6 feet, 2 inches tall and very handsome. He was even a model for Men's Wearhouse in Geneva, Illinois. He is sports oriented and played soccer, baseball, and track. On June 26, 2016, we invited Sam Anthony to join us for a family trip to Cooperstown, New York, where we would attend the state- and national-level baseball games that his younger brother Sean Michael would be pitching in. But he told us that he did not want to travel. His grandparents from his father's side also asked

Sam Anthony to go with them to a birthday celebration on July 2, 2016, but he declined that as well. His cousin Khristian, who was the same age, also nineteen years old, invited him to go for a Catholic Spiritual Retreat in Westchester on Saturday, July 3. Sam had three family invitations and refused all of them, not knowing that his life would completely change on July 3, that he would become disabled.

On July 2, Sam Anthony was already in bed at his grandparents' home by 8:30 PM.

when, one of his friends from school came to visit him and invited him to a bonfire birthday party in Aurora. Sam Anthony agreed to go. His friend drove that night and promised he would drive him back home early, since Sam Anthony had to work the following day at his summer job at a factory. Sam later told us he felt anxious for some reason within one hour of being at the party. He wanted to go home, but needed someone to take him back since he did not have a car or a driver's license at that time, and his home was about seven miles away from where the party was being held. No one wanted to do him a favor because it was too early, and he needed to enjoy the party. After midnight is when the accident happened.

The host's parents were inside while the boys and girls were outside. Though he was not the target of the random gunfire, my grandson was the only one among the ten or so others to get shot. He was then taken to the hospital for critical care. It was quite unfortunate.

Sam Anthony and the rest of the family did not want to cancel Nikalette's party, though. Sam Anthony told me to be with Nikalette at her party since so many other relatives and friends could be with him at the hospital. Nikalette's party had been planned for a year, and her brother did not want her to cancel her quinceañera celebration. Nikalette deserved everything that her mother and the rest of our family did for her for this party, since she was an outstanding student and a lovely young woman.

On the night of Nikalette's party, my mind was very preoccupied with my grandson's well-being. His condition was stable, but he was in intermediate care. I wanted to be his nurse, because I love all my family members and am always there for them, especially if they are sick. Nikalette was like my own daughter and she asked me to be with her on the day of her party. But at the same time, I also wanted to be with Sam Anthony. So I was physical present for Nikalette's party since I couldn't be in both places. Nikalette's quinceañera was well done (and she was happy and relieved that there was no more weekly dance practices!). But after the magnificent celebration for our princess Nikalette was over, we took time to care for Sam Anthony.

After several surgeries and nine months in and out of the hospital, Nikalette's brother had his leg amputated below the knee and finally got a suitable prosthesis after more than a year. In October 2018, he also went for another surgery to revise the stump to alleviate the pain.

CHAPTER II

Yabucoa, Puerto Rico, 2017

Nikalette entered the Puerto Rican beauty pageant in 2016. She had done a research paper on Yabucoa, Puerto Rico, where her father, Ramon, was born and raised, so she wanted to represent his town. She was motivated to learn everything about Yabucoa, PR. She asked me several times to take her to Puerto Rico, because she wanted to become familiar with her heritage. Nikalette, along with Khristian, Sam Anthony, and I, visited her father's town, on the beautiful island of Puerto Rico, for the first time in May 2017. I was happy to travel with my grandchildren.

Nikalette tried to encourage Sam Anthony to join us for this trip, even though he would need to travel by wheelchair after his left-leg amputation. Nikalette had a very close relationship with Sam Anthony; he was her role model in academics and sports. She played almost all the same sports that her older brother did, but their favorites were soccer and track. They helped each other. Sam Anthony assisted her with practices and enhancing skills, while she helped him with his recovery from the gunshot. His cousin Khristian helped Anthony with transfers to the wheelchair and helped him with self-care activities as needed. The two of them got a large room with equipment for a disabled person on the first floor in a nice motel, while Nikalette and I stayed in an apartment on the second floor in San Juan. The apartment belonged to a very close friend, Margarita Marchan Mankus, a well-known attorney in Illinois who was born and grew up in San Juan. Nikalette admired Margarita and loved to talk to her; she always told me, "I love her Puerto Rican accent!" We also rented a car to visit the beach, parks, and the rest of the island.

Nikalette's Research Paper on Yabucoa

The town of Yabucoa is located in the southeast part of Puerto Rico. This is the town where my father was born and raised. He died when I was only less than a year old, so I do not remember him, but I am so proud to call him my father. I am proud to be representing his hometown Yabucoa.

During my research for this paper, I learned a lot of interesting things. Yabucoa has a few different names such as Azucareros, Ciudad Del Nuevo Amanacer, and La Ciudad Del Azúcar. It was originally known as "Tierra de Agua" or Land of Water by Natives Indians that lived in this region before it was called Yabucoa. The patron for the city is Santos Angeles, The Holy Angels.

The shield that depicts the angels hold represents travelers and refers to the angels being the guides to the people on their journey here on earth. The canes have a guajana flower which represents the wealth of sugar cane, and the last the green land represents the fertile valley. The land is very fertile and is covered in crops of various kinds, such as sugar cane, tobacco, and plantain. It is surrounded by hills of San Lorenzo Batholith on three sides and by the Caribbean Sea on the fourth side. Yabucoa is divided into ten neighborhoods; Spanish town words called barrios: Aguacate, Calabaza, Camino Nuevo, Guayabota, Jacanas, Playa Guayanes, Tejas, Humacao, Yabucoa Pueblo, and finally my father's town Limones. After the Spanish colonization the region of Yabucoa belonged to Humacao, southeast of Puerto Rico.

I recently visited Yabucoa, and I even got to meet the mayor there. His name is Rafael Surillo, and he was genuinely nice and helpful. He was incredibly happy to hear that I would be representing Yabucoa. He gave me information about the history of the town as well.

I learned that the whole region that is now known as Yabucoa used to belong to the Taino Indians. The region of Guayaney was what it was known as, and their leader's name was cacique Guaraca. They were known as nice people but they had an enemy tribe called Caribe.

The Caribe, however, joined forces with them in order to fight off the Spanish colonization. They failed and the region joined forces with them in order to fight off the Spanish Colonization. Yabucoa then belonged to Humacao, and it was used for cattle and farming. It was not until later on October 3, 1793, that Don Manuel Colon de Bonilla and his wife Catalina Morales Pacheco donated the lands to the people and it became known as the town of Yabucoa.

The name Yabucoa was a Taino Indian term meaning "the place cassava is grown." The Taino believed in many gods and believed that being in the good graces of their gods protected them from disease, natural disaster, and war.

They would serve cassava bread, tobacco, and beverages to their gods as an offering. They even had ceremonial ballparks, a universal language, and the creation of religious cosmology. They had a hierarchy of deities whom they believed lived in the sky. Some of their language was copied by Europeans, such as Bohio or Strawhut, Hamaca also known as Hammock, and Maracas the musical instrument. This history still has an impact on Yabucoa today. There is a place called white stone in Spanish, Piedra Blanca, which looks like a pyramid from far away. It is dark and cold inside but is a stream of water there.

There are pots, utensils, and chairs made of stone inside. They were left there from when natives lived there, and they are so heavy nobody has moved them. Some believe it was a place for religious rites, and this belief gave it the other nickname of Convent ("El Convento" in Spanish). There is so much to see and to do in Yabucoa. For example, it has five beaches. One of them is called Dead Dog Beach because when the people cannot afford their dogs or find strays, they drop them off on this beach.

The dogs also breed there, so it becomes overpopulated. I do not recommend visiting this beach unless you are looking for a pet. There are, however, many other beautiful places to visit and places for entertainment as well. They have a public skate park, many sports arenas, a house of culture, and the Hacienda Santa Lucia ruins. There are many hotels and restaurants to stay at and eat at as well. Yabucoa is a great place to visit. They have many festivals there throughout the year. Some of the main ones are the sugar cane festival, Carmen festival, Quebradillas festival, Patron Celebrations, compassion festival (in Spanish Festival de la Compassion), and Mortorell Jibaro festival.

During these festivals they have criolla food, dancing, and entertainment of all kinds. It was so beautiful there I did not want to leave. As I said before, I am proud to be representing my father's hometown of Yabucoa. I have learned so much, and I cannot wait to go back and visit again. I recommended everyone to make the trip to see all that Yabucoa, Puerto Rico has to offer.

Yabucoa was a beautiful place to visit with warm weather, and the people were overly sweet and friendly, just like Nikalette. It was unfortunate to hear about Hurricane Maria, which almost destroyed all of Yabucoa in September 2017, just a few months after we visited.

Nikalette loved Puerto Rico. She said it was a beautiful island and wanted to return more often. She had family members in Yabucoa, but unfortunately, we did not have time to visit them. We visited museums, schools, hospitals, churches, the fire department, and the police department.

She felt confident about her research paper, and it was very well received by the Puerto Rican cultural council judges. In August 2017, Nikalette received recognition as Miss Congeniality and Miss Photogenic from the Aurora Puerto Rican Cultural Council. When she was sixteen, she was named Miss Yabucoa Puerto Rican 2017–2018 First Princess.

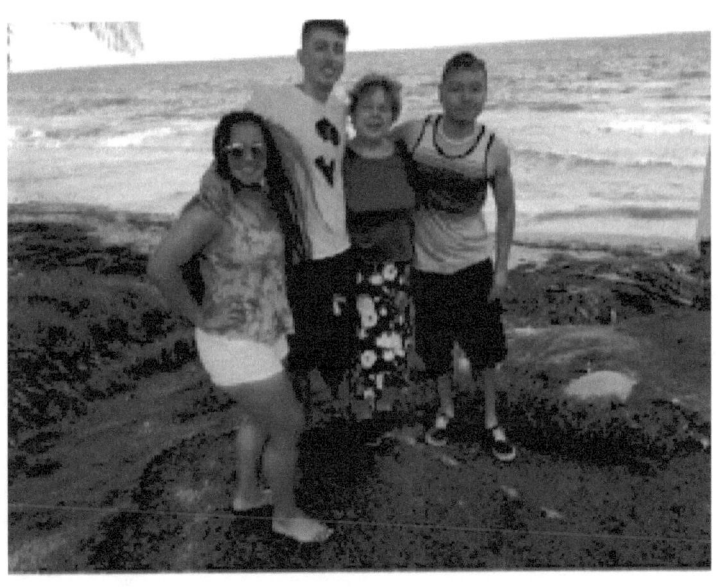

"Visiting Yabucoa, Puerto Rico: Nikalette, Sam Anthony, me, and Khristian, May 2017."

CHAPTER 12

Epilepsy: Medical and Nursing Overview

Epilepsy tends to produce repeated seizures due to abnormal brain cell activity, and it is a diverse condition that can be contributed to by varying genes with varied causes, etiologies, treatments, and prognosis. Living with epilepsy brings the risk of sudden, unexpected death. Research demonstrates that of one thousand people with epilepsy, one to two cases will experience death. In the United States, we have more than 20,000 cases per year. The treatment for epilepsy is assessed by a neurologist, and cases are classified by how seizures respond to certain anticonvulsants, which are prescribed by a neurologist.

A seizure is a sudden uncontrolled burst of electrical activity brief malfunction in the delicate structure of the brain, and when there is an imbalance between the excitatory and inhibitory forces in the brain, or cortical neurons, the seizure occurs. The nerve cells in the brain carry chemical and electrical messages from one part of the brain to another. There are more than twenty kinds of seizures, depending on which brain area is most affected. It is essential to know that all patients who have epilepsy also have seizures. Although not all people who have seizures have epilepsy.

Sleep activates the brain's abnormal electrical discharges at the cellular level within the central nervous system, which results in seizures for a person with epilepsy. Nikalette had seizure activity only during the night when she went to sleep. A person with this type of epilepsy will be unaware of the seizure but may develop headaches, drowsiness, behavioral changes, or anxiety after a seizure, in the postictal phase.

Seizures are so brief, and at times only careful observation or experienced medical personnel can detect them. Partial seizures are called now focal onset seizures. In my experience as a seasonal nurse working in neurology units at Rush University Medical Center, in Chicago Illinois, it was challenging to assess several types of seizures. While several of them were focal and then ended with grand mal seizures, or multiple seizures, other people suffered a fall without warning or aura. Other times patients went directly into grand mal seizure. At school, children with epilepsy can have seizures that are so brief they are only discovered by the teachers, nurses, babysitters, or the family. Though there may be a history of epilepsy in the family due to genetics, be aware that seizures can happen to any of us. Epilepsy can be genetic or acquired.

Types of seizures are as follows:

1. **Focal seizures.** These can start in one part of the brain. Symptoms can include a blank stare, chewing, smacking the lips, blinking the eyes for a moment, jerking, and loss of muscle tone before resuming normal activities. This may last a few seconds or longer. The patient does not know they are having a seizure. The seizure arises from a specific part of the hemisphere of the brain and is most common in children.

2. **Focal Onset Aware Seizures.** (Simple Partial Seizure) The patient is awake and aware of the seizure. Jerking begins in fingers or toes, then involves hands and arms, and at times they can have more seizures or this type of seizure can be an aura and to spreads to whole-body . These may last from seconds to minutes.

3. **Focal onset impaired awareness seizures.** These cause the person to become confused in their awareness; they used to be called a complex partial seizure. The symptoms include chewing, followed by random activity, and becoming unaware of surroundings; the person's actions become clumsy, not direct, and he or she may pick at clothing or pick up objects. These may last a few seconds to minutes.

4. General or grand mal seizures (tonic or clonic). These are the most serious and dangerous seizures; Nikalette experienced this type of seizure. These involve the entire brain. A seizure of this type may begin as a partial seizure at first, then ended up as a general or grand mal seizure. These seizures cause patients' bodies to become stiff and then to develop convulsions in the extremities, mouth secretions, body shaking, and problems breathing, leading to unconsciousness. These seizures can last from anywhere from two to five minutes. Emergency services should be called if needed. Postictal, the person may experience confusion and fatigue, followed by a return to full consciousness.

Generalize onset seizures and motor symptoms indicate a tonic seizure. The muscles will stiffen up, affecting the back, arms, and legs. If a person is standing, they may fall. and become unconsciousness. These seizures typically last fifty seconds to fourth minutes.

Clonic seizures involve rhythmical jerking muscle movements. Twitching affects the face, arms, and legs. The body flexes and extends repeatedly. There are mouth secretions and notable breathing difficulties. The seizure activity may last one to fourth minutes. You should stay with the person to prevent any injury, and call emergency services if needed. These types of seizures are dangerous.

5. Non-motor seizure. These usually include a behavior role arrest. This means that movement stops. These seizures don't involve muscle activity but do include emotions, thinking, and experiencing sensations. The person may stare into space with brief twitches at times without making any other movements.

6. Provoked and unprovoked seizures. Provoked seizures are secondary to trauma, the use of drugs such as cocaine, alcohol, or certain medications, drug withdrawal, lead poisoning, dehydration, alteration in blood sugar, or vitamin deficiencies, while unprovoked seizures are related to fever, infection, metabolic issues, genetics, Alzheimer's disease, brain progressive diseases such as tumors and aneurysms. Nikalette had a genetic predisposition related to her family history.

From my research, I found out that 2.5 million Americans are diagnosed with epilepsy. Around the world, sixty-five million have epilepsy. Worldwide, 5 to 10 percent may need surgery. Brain surgeries such as craniotomy are an option; these involve a surgical opening of the skull to provide access to dissecting tumors, clipping aneurysms, repairing cerebral injuries, and reducing seizures by removing the seizure focus. A neurologist may recommend craniotomy with advanced imaging technologies, allowing the surgical team to identify the seizure focus and remove a small tissue part of the brain, causing seizures to stop. It is a safe procedure when a patient is otherwise not responding to their anticonvulsant medications. It can reduce the severity and frequency of seizures or eliminate them altogether. Extensive preparation and post-operative care are needed. Of course, not everybody is a candidate for this surgery. Nikalette was not since she had a grand mal seizure, which involves all parts of the brain with seizure activity.

In the past, I worked in the neurology unit at Rush University Medical Center in Chicago, Illinois. I recall seeing several patients post craniotomy, and the procedure was highly beneficial for those patients. Their seizures decreased or stopped.

There are several types of craniotomies:

1. **Corpus callosotomy.** This surgical procedure interrupts the spread of seizures. The corpus callosum, which connects the left and right halves of the brain, is cut through to limit the spread of epileptic activity between the brain's two halves. It is also called a split-brain surgical procedure.

2. **Hemispherectomy.** This surgical procedure removes or disconnects the hemisphere that is least used and is the source of the seizures. This procedure helps to control seizures that come from one side of the brain.

3.**Multiple subpial transections.** This surgical intervention stops the seizure impulse by cutting nerve fibers in the outer layers of the brain's gray matter.

4. Temporal lobectomy. The most common type of surgery, this procedure removes a small part of the anterior temporal lobe that is causing the seizures, and significantly reduces or completes seizure control.

These surgical procedures are recommended only if the medication cannot otherwise control the seizures. However, as a nurse working closely with patients who had undergone these procedures, I did observe that most of them did very well as status postoperative.

The brain cells interact by electrical signals. A sudden robust amount of electrical energy affects all or part of the brain during a seizure. This affects the normal function of the brain due to seizure activity. Children with epilepsy are at risk for learning difficulties and depression. However, not everyone presents those symptoms, which at times is also part of the child's normal development independent of epilepsy and the treatment.

According to research, epilepsy can be developed at any age, but most are diagnosed in childhood. Two-thirds of children outgrow epilepsy by the time they are teens. In Nikalette's family history, her older brother from her father's side of the family used to have a similar type of nocturnal seizure, but his seizures stopped when he turned twenty-one. He is doing very well with no medications. We were all hoping that Nikalette's seizures would also end when she turned twenty-one. But every case is unique, and the treatment is individual.

Epilepsy affects the individual's life, family, and friends. It involves everyone's efforts to provide a safe environment to prevent injuries. There is a burden of care for caregivers of the person with seizures, especially not knowing when a seizure will occur.

Hospital Nursing Interventions Implementation

The nursing standards of care for Seizures Disorder are as follows:

1. Place patient on seizure precautions and maintain adequate respiratory and circulatory function. The nurse must stay with the patient with seizure activity and turn him on their side and provide a safety environment. Call for assistance if is needed.

2. Use ambu-bag and oxygen to assist patient breathing if as needed and side rails up three-from four. Side rails should be padded.

3. Have a suction machine ready. The patient may not handle their oral secretion and may aspirate; they may not be able to maintain their airway. Use oxygen and suction as needed.

4. Do not restrain the patient during seizure activity.

5. Do not put anything in their mouth during a seizure.

6. Assess, monitor, and describe seizure activity. First, what precipitated the seizure? Did the patient experience any pre-symptoms? Has the nurse observed that the patient would have pre- symptoms called an aura, such as a headache, nausea, and nervousness? (Note that not everyone has the same reactions.)

7. Nurse stays with the patient, observes the seizure activity, noting any rhythmic twitching, the specific part of the body, and the particular time of the seizure (such as 40 seconds, 2 or 3 minutes). Document the seizure activity and notify the MD.

8. Continue assessing the patient for the postictal phase; there are symptoms *after* the seizure activity as well. Document the observation. The nurse must document subjective and objective data. Offer emotional support to decrease anxiety level after the seizure as needed.

9. Educate patients and families about seizure precautions and medications to control seizures.

10. Medicate with anticonvulsants as prescribed per MD.

11. Encourage the patient to maintain and attend doctor appointments.

12. Keep the record of seizures and describe the seizure activity and the length of the seizure.

13. When positioning a person during a seizure, turn them on their side.

14. Place a video camera and noise alert in the patient's room.

15. Provide twenty-four-hour supervision if necessary.

16. Patient needs identification, such as a bracelet, for epilepsy.

Other Treatments for Epilepsy

Vagus nerve stimulation (VNS) is a small device implemented into the body through the left side of the chest; it's sometimes also called a pulse generator. This pulse generator is connected to a wire that attaches to the vagus nerve.

The vagus nerve is the most extended and complex of the twelve cranial nerves that transmit information to or from the brain to tissues and organs. The brain nerve bundles are neurons. They function by taking messages to and from the brain and other body parts. The vagus nerve has many paths in our body. One of them goes from the neck up to the brain. Vagus nerve stimulation is the therapy that takes this path from the neck to the brain to send electrical signals to prevent or shorten the length of seizures. Nikalette's close friend had a Vagus Nerve Stimulation, and she is doing much better. In fact, she was able to complete high school, and she attended Nikalette's funeral and other tribute ceremonies.

Risk Factors for Sudden Unexpected Death

The person is usually found dead in a prone position, lying on their stomach, as I found my granddaughter.

1. Not taking medications as prescribed. A proper dosage can prevent seizures or a drug overdose.

2. Status epilepticus. Having too many seizures at once is hazardous. Call emergency services immediately if the seizures do not stop.

3. Being alone. Not having someone nearby when having a seizure is dangerous.

Home Seizures: Precautions and Suggestions for Parents

1. Maintain a record of the seizures. Provide helmet to prevent head injury if needed, administer anticonvulsants as prescribed, follow recommendations from a doctor, and get routine blood tests. Electroencephalogram (EEG) and Magnetic Resonance Imaging (MRI) tests provide information to the doctors to diagnose epilepsy.

2. Lay your child down away from furniture, stairs, and sharp objects. Stay with the person and monitor seizure activity to provide a safe environment.

3. Place the person on their side to drain mouth secretions; seizures happen without warning.

4. Never restrain the person with seizure activity.

5. Place pillows on the floor if the patient tends to roll out of bed.

6. If you have a hospital bed at home, place the side rails up only three from four, and pad them.

7. Have the patient wear identification for seizure precautions.

8. Always keep the person's door open with their phone in reach.

9. Place a video camera and noise alert in the patient's room, which can then be monitored by their parents or primary caregiver.

10. Provide twenty-four hours supervision as needed.

11. Embrace new technology. Use a watch or smart band for epilepsy as a monitor.

12. Provide a counselor or psychologist as needed. (Nikalette had a counselor.)

13. If you travel to another country, look up the emergency phone number the first day you arrive, just in case it is needed.

14. Provide a trained seizure alert dog as needed if is needed

To prevent injuries or sudden death, we must implement seizure precautions.

Nikalette's Dreams

Nikalette had unfinished business; her dreams were gone instantly with her death. She had hoped to become a pediatric neurologist to help children with epilepsy and other brain diseases while bringing people close to the Lord. She was confident and tried to do profound studies in the medical field. She planned to take all advanced science and math classes; she was very proactive. She wanted to be prepared for her future. For that reason, she was going to join the Nurse Assistant Program in her last semester of high school in Fall 2018 to be able to gain knowledge and experience working at hospitals. She admired her doctors, pediatrician, and neurologist; they were all women, and Nikalette hoped to follow in their footsteps one day.

CHAPTER 13

Our Experience with Grief

I accept God's plan, and I thank him because I know my granddaughter's sudden death in her sleep ended her suffering with seizures. Still, today I am asking *why, why? Why does this happen to a very young person doing so many exceptional things in life?*

We said good-bye to Nikalette at the funeral home, which was incredibly sad. More than five hundred people came to her funeral. A friend said she counted one thousand. Many people told me they had to park their car more than ten blocks away from the funeral home. We welcomed all her teachers, classmates, and friends from her high school, her neurologist, and her nurse from Lutheran General Hospital in Park Ridge. Her pediatrician, Dr. Nadia, and other friends from Rush University Medical Center and Loyola University. Friends and family came from outside of Illinois: her older stepsister and stepbrothers came in from Tampa, Florida; her stepfather and other family members as well as aunts and uncles came from Dallas, Texas; and cousins and her aunt Madrina even flew in from Mexico. More than thirty hospital caregivers came from Loyola after work to pay their respects.

Nikalette's friends and classmates grieved with us. I hugged several students and listened to them. A while later, I went to the cemetery one day, and I found one of Nikalette's friends there crying. I hugged her and I began crying too. Then both of us started praying at Nikalette's gravesite until we could calm ourselves down and stop crying. Another time my husband found one of Nikalette's friends at the gravesite. She was talking to Nikalette and crying. Recently, I went to the gym. I found some of Nikalette's classmates there. They asked me to hug them. They cried and told me that they missed her a lot even though it had already been over two years since her passing. Another time I found two women at Nikalette's gravesite. I asked them if they knew my granddaughter. They said no; they told me they were driving around and saw so many fresh flowers. They decided to stop to visit this gravesite and they noticed red roses and the stone shaped like a heart, with pictures of Nikalette and the Virgin of Guadalupe. They told me she was an incredibly young and beautiful lady to have died. That gesture consoled me knowing that Nikalette is in heaven but still attracting people for good. They are grieving through faith in God. I found recently another family of two adults and three children vising Nikalette, I also asked them if they knew Nikalette; they said no but they stated, "We do come often to see her, because she was so young and beautiful."

Nikalette was very much loved, not only by me but by everyone who knew her. A compassionate young lady, she gave love to everybody, and she received love and respect in return.

The only way that I have found consolation and comfort for myself is by going to church daily or visiting Nikalette at the cemetery it was almost daily for the first year now is less often. The grieving process is like any other illness; our emotions are in overdrive. Grief is the last act of life we have to give to those we love and is a perfectly normal response to a loss. It also varies individually because we all react differently to a loss. Our personality, environment, culture, self-esteem, and past experiences all factor into our response. Our feelings about a critical change can be dramatic or nondramatic. It is normal to have any of these emotions. But you are not alone. We all suffer pain from the loss of our loved ones, from divorce, illness, loss of independence, or any other crisis in our lives. But we also need to understand that the sadder we feel and the longer we adhere to this emotional state, the harder it is to come out of it.

The traumatic loss of Nikalette sent me into deep emotional reactions that interfered with my ability to function normally. I learned that it is essential not to make any significant or critical decisions if we are experiencing grief after any death or tragic situation. However, I would not have survived this painful experience without my faith in my Lord. My faith is a gift from God.

"Thus faith comes from what is heard, and what is heard comes through the word of Christ."
Romans 10:17

After Nikalette's death, I had no energy in the initial days. I was unable to sleep or eat. I suffered immensely from Nikalette's absence in my life. I felt that Nikalette had been taken away from us too early in her life, at only seventeen years old. My husband and I were older and closer to going to be with our Lord than she was. I felt we should be the ones to die, not her.

Then in the first two weeks after Nikalette's funeral, I was in shock and denial for many days. I was very depressed. I would cry and cry, unable to sleep, eat, or do anything, and had no energy. When I went to daily Mass, I felt comforted when praying the rosary with family and friends. People came to pray together with us. We had about two hundred people in my house over the course of the first two weeks after the funeral. They brought us food and cakes, and they also shared memories of my granddaughter. It was comforting to know that Nikalette was extremely loved by her classmates, friends, and the community of Aurora. Nikalette always listened to them, brought them flowers on their birthdays, and provided emotional and spiritual support to her classmates when they needed it.

For me, the best way to honor Nikalette's memory was to draft this book about my warrior princess who battled epilepsy. Otherwise, I would just be crying and crying. Nikalette was like my own daughter; we did so many things together. She was always in my room asking questions regarding school or family or just coming in to talk. She would check in me or would say, "Good morning, Grandma! We need to pray" or "We need to go to the gym." Every time I remembered her, I would get very emotional. The Lord helped us to control this pain. I started going to Holy Cross Church in Batavia for the Eucharistic Adoration three times a day. Now I mostly go once a week, or wherever I can. I prayed daily and attended Mass at St. Rita Church, the Marmion Abbey in Aurora, or at Presence Mercy Hospital. Visiting the churches was very consoling. I felt desperate to go to a holy place and had a strong desire to attend Mass. I tried to keep myself busy, but I also did not want to answer the phone or talk to anyone. It was emotionally painful.

My deep faith in God helped me spiritually and emotionally. I accept God's plan and move forward. We can grow tremendously when we face a tragic event, such as losing a loved one in our lives. Even though it is painful, it still is a learning process. We become better people and grow closer to God by finding new coping mechanisms and new friends in similar situations. We can learn to adapt to our unique and painful situation. We will also better understand others who are still in the midst of facing similar problems; we will show them more compassion and empathy.

Now we are praying the rosary with my family and friends. I exercise more often. As a Catholic Christian, I believe that by accepting Jesus Christ as my Savior and asking God to forgive me my sins. I will be in heaven when I die with my Nikalette and other loved ones who have already departed. God has unconditional love for everyone. With repentance and acceptance of the Lord as our Savior, and practice our faith God will lead us to eternal life to be with our family members and friends who have died. But also, here in this world, our life is better in all aspects. The spiritual connection with God benefits those of us who honestly believe in him. At this moment, life is more difficult not only here but also around the world. So many things are uncertain as we are dealing with the COVID-19 pandemic, it did improve with the vaccines and there may be other viruses or world crises to come. We do not know, but with God, we will be victorious. I consider myself extremely optimistic, but I also have to be realistic.

As a registered nurse, every day before I went to work, I did daily Bible readings. I prayed to prepare myself for emergencies so I could function as an accountable and compassionate registered nurse at any hospital setting. I told all my family members to pray every day. Nikalette always said her prayers to me when I was not at work. I miss her a lot: my warrior princess, my queen, Nikalette. I used to call her my queen. And she loved it. Several people said that she looked like me. Others said Nikalette looked like her father's family. Either way, she was beautiful inside and out.

Stress Response: How Our Bodies React to Grief

I knew about the stress response affecting my body and mind, and I understood my symptoms because I am a nurse with experience. Grief increases multiple physical and mental symptoms. The release of chemical neurotransmitters and hormones internal in my body affected my health, and I just wanted to cry and cry for hours then I started praying. Nikalette, to me, was like my daughter.

In grief, our brain acts abnormally and releases several neurochemicals and hormones, causing a disruption to our health. More stress neurotransmitters increase due to the body's overreacting to the tragedy. Neurotransmitters send messages from one nerve cell to another; there are billions of chemicals in the central nervous system. They pass information, carry, boost, and balance signals between neurons and other cells throughout the body; too much or too little will affect us physically and mentally. Symptoms are individual; we all react differently to tragic events. But it is essential to maintain good health to adapt to new situations. So my question was *how can I improve myself?* I was dealing with grief and with symptoms of depression, such as a loss of appetite, inability to sleep, and no energy.

I knew my cortisol level was off because my concentration and problem-solving skills were vastly diminished, making me prone to anxiety and depression. I honestly could not function as a mother, wife, or nurse immediately after Nikalette died. I needed to take care of myself physically, mentally, and spiritually. At times, we as a family experienced outburst of emotion: anger, crying, or insomnia for countless hours or even days. After the tragic event, I did encourage my family members to verbalize their feelings. I also told them, "Cry if you need to cry."

I wanted to present myself as strong and healthy in front of my family and friends because I tried to console them. Still, at times, I was unable to do it. I did remind them to listen to their feelings to let their emotions out of their systems before they could affect them with more serious physical or mental symptoms. For example, I experienced high sadness, negative thinking, inability to sleep, depression and anxiety, and gastrointestinal symptoms including nausea, vomiting, and lack of appetite. All of these can lead to a decrease in our immune system. That means we open our bodies to other illnesses and problems with our health. So please, if you are grieving, see your doctors or other experts if you need them.

I walked and exposed myself to the sunshine to calm down; getting vitamin D from the sunlight is the best for our health. According to researchers, that's a good way to stimulate the internal production of chemical neurotransmitters to preserve our health.

Tryptophan, an amino acid, builds protein for body function; in our brains, it is converted to serotonin, which relaxes our muscles and helps us feel better. Tryptophan is found in foods such as chicken, fish, eggs, milk, chocolate, and bananas. Unsurprisingly, those were my favorite foods. L-Tryptophan must be supplied to our diet.

Melatonin, which helps us sleep, is a natural hormone released in response to darkness and suppressed by light. So we should always sleep in a dark room so we can get good rest.

Dopamine is a brain neurotransmitter which coordinates our body movement and makes us feel better. This chemical neurotransmitter rewards our brain by telling us we did a good job. So, if you have time to volunteer, you will get a dose of dopamine. You will feel better and have a good positive attitude, just as Nikalette did. As a family, we did continue volunteering in our community after this tragic event. Helping others with kindness improves our health. Having a more positive feeling about ourselves, such as when we accomplish a task or receive something pleasurable like good news, is so helpful.

Serotonin, dopamine, norepinephrine, and gamma-aminobutyric acid (GABA) are those neurotransmitters that regulate our body's mood and anxiety levels. Neurotransmitter levels are constantly changing internally because of stress, which is a normal response, especially when dealing with a tragic event. Research has found that grief leads to endocrine, immune, autonomic nervous, and cardiovascular problems. It is very dangerous to remain in depression for longer time if you are having similar symptoms as I was, please see your primary doctor.

I decided to relieve my symptoms of depression caused by grieving. My physical symptoms included gastrointestinal upset, headaches, insomnia, and mood changes. I knew the chemicals in my body and brain were totally off, which was a normal reaction due to my deep pain and stress. I talked to my family, friends, and coworkers, which helped to bring relief from emotional pain. I also walked daily or swam at the gym near my home.

When we exercise, our brain produces other chemicals and neurotransmitters to help us feel better. Several of them are beneficial, especially when we are facing a loss. My family members attended psychotherapy for a few sessions. Those activities were helpful to my family and me. This is important because psychotherapy helps to convert your sad and negative thinking and behavior patterns into healthier ones.

Additional Brief Descriptions of Neurotransmitters

1. Serotonin is a neurotransmitter. If we exercise and have positive thoughts, a higher intake of healthy foods helps improve our mood.

2. Glutamate and GABA (gamma-aminobutyric acid) are the major neurotransmitters in the brain. They work together to control and balance the brain. They also have a calm and relaxing effect. They help memory and learning. Sources of glutamate include tomatoes, corn, cow milk, bananas, fruits, cheese, and chocolate.

3. Endorphins are opioid neuropeptides that help control pain and emotions and improve mood. Suppose we exercise thirty minutes daily (whether aerobic or anaerobic exercise); researchers have found that this will relieve both pain and depression.

4. Dopamine helps the body move, control motor functions, and reward behavior with positive feel-

ings. Being kind to others, exercising, and volunteering will improve our health.

5. Cortisol is a stress hormone and also a neurotransmitter. Symptoms of high cortisol are fatigue, headache, hypertension, and irritable behavior. We need to relax and exercise more often, three to five times a week for thirty to forty-five minutes. This was certainly helpful to us as a family as a way to feel better.

6. Epinephrine, also called adrenaline, is a hormone and neurotransmitter in the body. Adrenaline is released by the adrenal glands located on top of the kidney. The primary function is to increase cardiac output, increase heart rate, and raise glucose levels.

7. Norepinephrine and epinephrine both cause feelings of alertness involved in the body's fight or flight response, helping us act in times of danger or stress. The brain sends signals to stimulate the autonomic nervous system. The sympathetic and parasympathetic nervous system drives the fight and flight response, which can last sixty seconds as a response to acute stress. All this happens inside of our bodies. We'll only notice the symptoms.

*

I did not have an appetite. I forced myself to eat vegetables. I also ate high protein foods such as milk products, eggs, fish, and chicken. Along with occasional ice cream with chocolate cake, I made sure to eat fruits, drink plenty of fluid, take vitamins, and exercise daily. I also took a sleeping pill because I had insomnia. It is essential to maintain good health. If you are facing a similarly painful situation, see your healthcare provider.

All my symptoms were the standard response to grieving. However, emotional pain can arise due to many other traumatic events in our lives, such as losing a job, getting divorced, experiencing the death of a pet, moving out of our house, getting sick, dropping out of school, or losing our independence.

For three to four weeks, grief also affected my cognition, emotions, and behavior. The symptoms included nightmares, uncertainty, intrusive images, suspicion, blaming others, poor attention, problems with concentration, decreased awareness, and hypervigilance. My family and I also experienced difficulties concentrating, increased worry, and insufficient attention. Luckily those symptoms only lasted for the first two weeks.

My family all experienced different symptoms. I experienced fear, guilt, anxiety, apprehension, emotional outbursts, depression, shock, denial, and panic. I used to cry and cry by myself; sometimes I was not able to stop. Other times we all cried together, or we shared stories about Nikalette. We laughed too at times when we looked at her pictures or remembered joyful times spent together.

I experienced withdrawal, inability to rest, intensified pacing, walking more to attempt to clear my mind, and changes in communication. I did not want to answer the phone or socialize. I had those symptoms for three to four weeks. A few members of my family also had to see a doctor, particularly my daughter Sandy, Nikalette's mother. If you are facing a similar situation and have many of these symptoms, please consult your physician for evaluation and medical treatment.

The grieving process includes denial, anger, bargaining, depression, and acceptance. But the grieving process does not happen in order. We all have different needs and different coping skills. Our reaction to crises is influenced by our genetics, environment, support system, friends and family, and our experiences from the past. In my own experience, I was in denial at first, then moved on to bargaining, depression, and acceptance. However, at times, I remember activities that we did together with Nikalette and I thanks God for those memories.

*

On August 14, 2018, only three months after Nikalette's passing, I lost my sister due to septicemia after a kidney transplant that was very difficult time for me and my family I did attended her funeral services in Mexico but I was not able to stop crying, I still feel the loss of my granddaughter and now my sister that was very devastated I was very close to my sister, but was very comforting to pray daily with all my family and friends. Then a coworker, a young nurse, died unexpectedly on October 16, 2018. (I did not attend her memorial service because I was at the hospital taking care of my grandson Sam Anthony who needed stump revision for his stump in his left leg secondary to severe pain and problems with his prothesis.) Then on December 20, 2018, a lifelong friend died from heart problems. I also attended his funeral. It was very depressing he was like a brother to us we travel with his wife to Alaska ,Cancun, and many other places we socialized with all his grown daughters and our family too a lot of activities together. This was all the same year after Nikalette's death.

On December 26, 2019, I attended the funeral services for Father Gerardo Manuel Gomez Reza. a young priest from St. Rita's church who died approximately in five weeks with recently diagnostic with cancer. I was not able to stop crying at each funeral. Nikalette and the whole rest of our family had a good relationship with Father Gerardo Manuel. He did many religious ceremonies for our family, including the funeral mass for my granddaughter and the Rite of committal(Burial or interment) at the funeral home and at the cemetery. We did pray the rosary at the funeral home and short Scriptural verse and Father Gerardo Manuel was leading us with those prayers. He is in heaven and we thanks God that he was a very dedicated and compassionate priest; we all miss him.

I was living in a dream for a few days after each funeral. I revived everything from each funeral that I attended. I knew that if I chose to stay in that state for long periods by not accepting the reality of the situation, it would cause me to be in so much pain. I would have the potential for physical and psychological problems for the rest of my life.

I also experienced anger by pushing away people, making excuses, behaving inappropriately, and withdrawing to avoid the pain. I refused to answer the phone for about four months. I was so angry that I was not able to save Nikalette after so many years of nursing experience, and then I lost others five lovely people who I was very attached to. All of them were gone in a very short period of time, only eighteen months.

Dealing with the anger was difficult for me due to my feelings of guilt, constantly asking myself what I could have done to prevent the loss of my Nikalette. I was bargaining with God. I felt better by attending daily mass and putting everything in my Lord's hands. The new situation required me to calmly let go of the losses from the past, and now I accepted and moved forward.

According to the literature, some people are so resilient that they can recover from grief in a short period. Somehow others will be trapped, and they may not come out from their loss. My experience took me longer than two to three years. Still, in one year in six months, I lost five lovely, charming people. And I could not recuperate from so much emotional pain. But finally, I am able to enjoy life again now, and return to work and socialize I thought to myself *without God in my life, I would not survive.*

I did go through all the steps of the grieving process. My Lord Jesus Christ gave me strength and faith to continue on and finally accept this painful period when I had to say good-bye to five dearest family and friends. May they rest in peace with our Lord and for me accept the plan of God and learn to live again by returning to work, spend time with my family and friends and help others.

Our Intervention for Grieving

We as a family had counseling sessions two to three weeks after the funeral with Rev. Msgr. Robert J. Willhite. My daughter also attended a session with a social work counselor and a support group. We were appreciative of their time and kindness; we also saw our regular doctor. At times, our self-care was neglected. So, we also needed to go for a manicure, pedicure, and massage. We prayed as a family together, cried together, and listened to each other. We had dinners as a family and with Nikalette's classmates and friends. I joined another interfaith group at St. Rita church for additional spiritual support to maintain my emotional well-being.

It is reported in the research literature that people can die due to grieving that is unresolved, if they are unable to manage themselves or not able to function as an average person. According to research, other symptoms of unresolved grief include either the inability to sleep or sleeping for much more than eight to ten hours, gastric distress, lack of appetite, anxiety, anger, frustration, and short temper. We can be forever in this stage if we choose to stay in denial, shock, or depression, which is unhealthy because all the brain chemicals are being depleted. Depression can lead to unresolved grief, which in turn can lead us into maladaptive behaviors and addictions such as overeating, gaming, smoking, drinking alcohol, shopping, and taking drugs such as cocaine or other stimulants. As an experienced nurse, I suggest seeing your doctor, or a counselor, if you are in a similar situation, attending church and giving everything to the Lord. I suggest exercise, doing community service, and following a healthy diet. Find new friends at church. It is extremely difficult to adapt to a new situation after hardship, so please stay connected to God, family, friends, community and return to work.

It isn't easy to take the first step, even just to make the appointments. I was not myself during this time. I cried until no more tears came out. It was a sorrowful time. The only thing that was a big help for my family and me was to pray the rosary daily and attend Mass more often. As a nurse, I did feel that I needed to move forward. I did not want to heal partially. I needed to heal holistically: body and mind, physically and spiritually.

I wanted to heal so I could comfort and support others and continue working as a volunteer nurse. I remember when Nikalette told us to be stronger because God loves all of us: that was one of her favorite statements. She used this statement with her classmates, friends, and family. It is comforting to know that Nikalette was teaching her classmates to be close to God for us to be successful in life.

If we do not heal from loss, or any other critical incident, we deal with incomplete grief. Writing this book in both language English and Spanish was helping me to heal because it is very therapeutic to write my own experience. I never wrote a book so it has been a challenge I was scam since I did not know what I was doing with so much pain now. I am doing the processes myself to publish this book. I pray that I am also able to assist others who are going through a similar experience and to honor the memory of our warrior princess.

When there is no support system, family, or friends, it is hard to go through the grieving process alone. We need to be with people who are positive and helpful. I stayed away from negative toxic people to preserve my health, especially when I was in so much emotional discomfort. To this day, I am overly sensitive whenever I attend a funeral. Three years after the death of my granddaughter, my sister, two friends, and our priest, but nothing compared to the first months of grieving. I thought I was dreaming; I was highly emotional.

It was excruciating going to so many funerals. I attended all those funeral services and could not stop crying because I remembered Nikalette's funeral. I ran to church to attend mass and just to be a sacred and peaceful place with our Lord. I want you, the reader, to know that staying connected with God, family and friends is essential. Be self-aware of your thoughts and feelings, attend church, or join any other support groups; please do not isolate yourself because you suffer more you need a friend to hold your hand to listen to you feelings and to walk with you through any difficult time.

We can grow tremendously when we face a tragic and painful event. The completion of this book in my second language and also in Spanish plus doing an in-depth review of the epilepsy literature enriched not only my brain with wisdom but also my whole experience of these events.

I desire to continue as a volunteer in my nursing profession, in my church, and in my community involvement, and to be deeply connected with family and friends, as Nikalette was. She made an impact and now she is continuing to do so through this book.

As a Catholic Christian, I believe in accepting Jesus Christ as my savior and asking God to forgive me my sins with repentance and going to confession with our priest, doing penance practicing our faith by serving others. Our Lord Jesus Christ will lead us to eternal life to be with our family members and friends who have departed this world. But also, here in this world, He makes our lives better in all aspects. The spiritual connection with God benefits all of us who honestly believe in our Lord. I do respect any religious beliefs and admire people with strong faith. But I do feel very sorry when people are facing grief alone. To me this tragic experience lead me to honor Nikalette's memory by writing her biography in English and Spanish.

CHAPTER 14

Nikalette's Last School Assignments

Nikalette wrote a paper for her Junior English Class # 200. Her teacher was Mrs. Sheila McQuade. Here is what she wrote a month before her departure to heaven. Nikalette's assignment was to analyze a quote that influenced her.

Setting a goal and being determined to reach it without letting anything or anyone get in your way is a successful sacrifice.

Many people think quitting or giving up makes things easier. At the end of the day, it really makes you struggle, so once you start something, you always must finish it!

This quote, "IT IS HARD TO BEAT A PERSON WHO NEVER GIVES UP," portrays how you will never be defeated because of how far you have come.

When you have something in mind and work hard to achieve it, you feel satisfied and proud of yourself. This quotation affects my philosophy of life by reminding me not to give up and to always stay strong and finish strong, not just education-wise but athletic-wise too. All of this proves how hard it is to work and what results in you will get in the end for always being dedicated.

It strengthens your mindset and how you view things.

Being positive is another good strategy for helping with your responsibilities as you get older.

When you are always being respectful and positive, good things happen.

In addition, when you show people, you have the strength to finish and not to give up, they start to have faith in God and you, which builds up your confidence and worth.

Having goals to achieve, faith in God by your side, and determination will get you through any struggle in the world.

This quote shows that no one can compete with you or even take you down; once you are noted as a dedicated person, you will forever reach the destination of your goals in life.

This quote reflects how I am as a person; I will never give up no matter what distractions come my way.

I will realize how far I have come and know how to keep on going. I will continue to work hard and give my best efforts towards obstacles with my health, sports, academics, or just reality.

She also wrote a personal essay that she could have potentially sent with her college application. It was done May 4, 2018, just six days before she died from the seizure. It was done for her HOSA English class.

Personal Statement Essay: Hello, my name is Nikalette Rivera Simental. I am 17 years old and a current student at West Aurora High School. I am an outgoing, determined, and passionate person who loves to get involved. Now to start off, I would like to inform you of some hobbies and unique qualities about me. I am a cross-country runner here at West Aurora High School, and when I am not running, I am usually at the gym working out. Besides going to the gym, I love to stay active and travel. I have so far been to Canada, Florida, Mexico, New York, Puerto Rico, Tennessee, and Texas.

I plan to continue traveling and experiencing new different things throughout the next couple of years. I am also a Link Leader and Student Assistant. A Link Leader is an individual who helps freshman and sophomore students get involved in afterschool curricula. To assist them in making sure they feel welcome and finally help them with any academic classes. I am also part of the HOSA Academy, which is an academy for any students who are planning to go into the medical field in the future.

Furthermore, I am graduating a semester early from high school and getting my certified nurse assistant in the fall. My future goals for myself are extremely high, and I am determined to reach them. If you have not noticed yet, I am a person who never gives up and always finishes what I start. One of my favorite quotes that relate to my running athleticism is "In order to win the race, you've got to be in the race." I hope to maintain a good spirit and continue working hard through all the obstacles that come along the way.

Additionally, this past summer, I was in a pageant here in Aurora, Illinois. I was running against two other girls to be Miss Puerto Rico of Aurora. My father, who has been deceased since I was less than one year old, he was 100% Puerto Rican. I never got to meet him or make memories with him. So, to make him proud of me, I decided to join the pageant and research information about his town. During this process, I learned new things and volunteered at many events.

On top of that, I got to go to Puerto Rico for the first time. When I went there, it was the best experience of my life. I felt so welcome and was treated like a queen. The most amazing part was when I went to the police department of my father's town, Yabucoa. I told them I was currently running for a pageant in Illinois to try to and become Miss Yabucoa, Puerto Rico.

Once I revealed that to them, they had taken me to meet the Mayor of Yabucoa. His name is Rafael Surillo. He was nice and very welcoming. After that, the police officer took my family and me on a road trip up to the mountains. As soon as we got to the top, you could see the whole view of Yabucoa.

It was an extremely beautiful and unforgettable moment. Until this day, I thank the Lord for that memorable blessing. When it came to an end, I did not want to leave the gorgeous island of mine. It was the hardest thing I have done. Only because

I felt so welcomed and the view was stunning. Finally, I wrote a research paper about Yabucoa and the wonderful visit I went on. On the day of the pageant, I was nervous and excited at the same time. I was rewarded Miss Photogenic and Miss Congeniality.

Overall, I ended up winning Miss Puerto Rico Princess 1 of Aurora, Illinois, and it was the greatest experience ever. Although it was stressful and a lot of work, I made it through by pushing myself and always finishing what I had started. It contained plenty of dedication, confidence, effort, and time. Today since I am the Princess, I get to be on a float in the Puerto Rican Parade and Festival of Downtown Aurora coming up this summer. Without all the hard work and determination, I would never have been able to finish the competition. The goals in life are to succeed, learn, and experience new things, have fun, and never give up on things you put your mind to.

With God, all things are possible.

Nikalette respected and admired Mrs. Sheila McQuade, her HOSA English teacher. She spoke very highly about all her teachers, but especially Mrs. Sheila McQuade and Mrs. Smith, her chemistry teacher. She told me she learned a lot from them both.

CHAPTER 15

Procession

November 1 and November 2 are days for our Spanish culture to celebrate the life of the people who are now with the Lord in heaven. On November 1, 2018, at 5 pm, Nikalette's family, classmates, and friends celebrated Nikalette's life. We visited Nikalette's gravesite, a peaceful area at the cemetery at Sugar Grove, Illinois.

We had a procession from our home in Sugar Grove to the cemetery, which is about one mile from my house. Most of us walked with a candle to remember Nikalette. My friend Claire Perez, religious leader for the Rite of Christian Initiation of Adults from Saint Rita of Cascia in Aurora, Illinois, was asked to prepare this ceremony. She initiated prayers at Nikalette's gravesite. Every prayer was translated into Spanish as a tribute to Nikalette and comfort all of us. She also read

Romans 14:7–8: "None of us lives for oneself, and no one dies for oneself. For if we live, we live for the Lord, and if we die, we die for the Lord; so then whether we live or die, we are the Lord's."

The prayers and songs emphasized that we needed to believe and trust in Jesus Christ as Nikalette did. We all cried and cried as if we had just buried her. It had only been six months since her departure to heaven. Nikalette's memories and her spirit were with us. The Lord is love, and trust in Him sustained us through this difficult time.

After this ceremony at the cemetery, we went to Prestbury Clubhouse. We had dinner with beef, chicken, pizza, rice, pasta, vegetables, cookies, and fruits. We had time for reflection with Nikalette's classmates, family, and friends. They read poems and shared memories about Nikalette. We had pictures and decorations to honor her memory and the memories of other family members who are in heaven. In the Mexican culture, on November 1, we celebrate the saints. People who have died before they turn eighteen years old are considered angels of God.

On November 2 Mexico celebrates the Day of the Dead, Dia de los Muertos in Spanish. It is a holiday celebrated throughout Mexico, Central America, and South America. In those regions, they celebrate with altars to remember the dead with their pictures, flowers, music, and favorite dishes. Mexico DF, celebrate the Day of the Dead with a enormous parade. We honored this day to remember Nikalette's life and accomplishments.

The following poems were by provided by a few family members and friends:

Optimism Poem

By Grandparents Juan and Lilia Simental

Forgive yourself for past mistakes, your weakness, failures, and do not waste your time thinking about the past with negative experiences, the past is gone.

Life is too short; pray daily, develop a close relationship with God, have faith in our Lord, practice your faith by serving others and be positive, focus in the moment.

Realize your imperfections, and remove barriers, do not limit yourself you are perfect with the love of God.

Discover your possibilities, talents, find your purpose in life, and value life.

Make a new friend, love God first, love yourself, and love others even with difficult personalities.

Accept responsibility for your actions and improve the task.

Dream one big dream for your future.

It may come through; for God, it is not impossible. Imagine yourself floating in space happy, extremely happy.

Watch the sunset, the rain, the snow, the trees, flowers and enjoy them.

Cherish, and have gratitude for what you have.

Cherish who you are, cherish that you can see, eat, you can swallow and walk with God and the loved ones at your side.

You are a valuable person, an especially important human being with a purpose and a mission to accomplish in life.

God is with you. Help others who need you, listen, have an I-can-do attitude with compassion.

Treat everybody with respect and dignity the way you want to be treated.

Be happy with what you have; life is short. It was noticeably short for Nikalette.

Nikalette wanted all students, families, and friends to be successful.

She used to tell them to perform well in school, sports, or job, and learn a healthy way to deal with grieving, learn precautions with epilepsy, and be involved in your community.

Live your life to its fullest, love the Lord and others as if today will be our last day; do not judge, only my Heavenly Father is to judge us.

Poem and Reflection

By Cristy Sims, Nikalette's aunt

My spirit and the Lord's spirit will always be with you.

From Nikalette our angel in heaven: my spirit and the Lord's spirit will always be with you. Everything is fine; I am in heaven with all the saints, angels, and family, friends that are with our Heavenly Father. I want my family, friends, teachers, coaches, counselors, doctors, and all people who came in contact with me to laugh and smile as we did in the past. Please continue to enjoy your time as we enjoyed ours together. One day we eventually will be reunited in heaven with our Lord Jesus Christ.

My life is not gone; it is transformed. My spirit still is with you as long you do not forget me. I will always live with our memories. I want you to know that I am not in pain. No sorrow, no apprehension, no fears, no seizures. Everything here is peaceful, safe, love, with beautiful gardens, brilliant, clear, no darkness.

The brightness is everywhere. I am with Jesus Christ our Lord.

Nothing that I lived with all of you was in vain. Everything has a value. Continue doing good, my lovely family, my classmates and friends, and my community. Each day immerse yourself in God's presence, enhance and strengthen your faith. We are here today. We do not know about tomorrow. Only our Creator is in charge of our lives. So you will not suffer the day you pass away, stay firm with the Lord; He will open His arms for you as He opened His arms to me. He loves all of us, no matter where you have been, your race, or your gender. God has unconditional love for all of us, as long you repent and accept Him as your Savior, our Heavenly Father, our Lord Jesus Christ. He will be bringing us together one day. For now, have strong faith in Him. Nothing will make you happy, only God and your God's family. Allow your life to shine in peace, love, and hope so others will notice the brightness in your face given by God, as He gave everything to me and others who trust him.

Remember me the way I was before I went to the Lord, peacefully now for eternal life.

The day that you come to the Lord, do not fear. I want you to fly as I did, fly higher than myself; I will wait for you at the door of our Lord's home. Where it is a very peaceful, spiritual place with beautiful stars, lights, green gardens, all the angels and saints, your family and friends. Who is in heaven with Jesus Christ? It is not pain or suffering, no seizures anymore.

Maria Jose Garcia was a close friend of Nikalette's from middle school until Nikalette died. She presented this beautiful poem to one hundred classmates and family members on March 9, 2019, as we celebrated Nikalette's eighteenth birthday at Sandy's house surrounded by Nikalette's photos, poems, and cheeriest memories. We all cried after this presentation.

Nikalette, your well-placed chin,

Your cute little nose,

The way you would blossom like a rose,

The perfect smile of yours

That would end all kinds of wars.

Your long sleek hair that would touch the jeans that.

You would always wear and the loud continuous laugh.

I would give up anything to hear you laugh to make us happy.

Now all I have are videos and photographs.

I try to not shed a single tear.

I know you are still here.

However, sometimes it is hard.

Because I have the memory of you inside me, scarred,

We will always remember May 10 because that is when our world turned grey.

We question God why you could not just stay, but instead we let go and pray.

As we all try to move on, nothing will replace the fact that you are gone.

Please God, protect Juni, Janessa, Cesar, Raquel, Jordan, Angelina, Anthony, and Sean, and other family members, classmates, and friends.

Heal the beating heart of your Mother Sandy because she will always love you like no other.

In addition, forgive us if you see us cry, we are just sad we did not get to say good-bye.

As we set you free to fly, we'll remember to keep our heads high because now we have.

Angel in the sky and heaven

Please be strong in your faith, you must not paralyze yourself.

Do it now, we are here temporally?

Eternal life is with the Lord.

When you completed you work then

The Lord will gently call you home.

Safely home with all the angels, saints, family, and friends who already went to the Lord and earned eternal life. Nikalette is gone to heaven but not forgotten.

CHAPTER 16

Consolation Letters from Family and Friends

Here is a letter to Nikalette from Angelina, her younger sister.

April 2019

Dear Nikalette:

I know that I may not have been the best sister, and I am sorry for that, but I want you to know that I will always love you and treasure every moment we had together. I wish we could create more memories together, but I hope you know that I miss you and love you so much forever. You mean the world to me, and you will always be on my mind, and I hope you know that. I will never forget about you because you were the best sister that anyone could ever have. You were smart, beauti-

ful, and kind. I love you so much, and I miss you a lot.

I know that I do not talk about you often, but it is because I know you are still with us in your spirit. You are in a better place with Jesus Christ. Nikalette, you are our angel in heaven now. I hope one day I can see you again, but for now I will always have beautiful memories and the pictures reminding me of our time together.

Nikalette, I admired you because you were very spiritual, creative, a strong leader, loving, and had an amazing attitude. You helped us with homework and chores for the house. You were a great role model. You are the best sister, and I love you so much, and I miss you a lot. I would never change anything about you.

Nikalette, you were a kind sister and friend to me. I remember your precious laugh when you used to mess around with me and Sean, our brother. I loved spending time with you and going to places with you and hanging out with you and our family. I will never forget how you always asked me to sleep in the same room with you because of your seizures. Or the time we went to the gym, and you took Sean and me with you. I admired your confidence that you had in everything, in school, sports, church, community work, volun-

teering with the homeless, and Easter celebrations.
I loved it when we would all have dinner together
as a family making great memories.

Nikalette, it has been extremely hard for me not
to have you here at home. You are my only sister, and
I miss you so much. You are the one I used to talk
to about everything. You were always there guiding
me and always by my side. Now I am sad that I no
longer have a sister here to talk to like I used to. You
always listened to me and spent time with me. You
never teased me or made fun of me when I told you
about my feelings like other people used to.

It's as though no one cares about my feelings as
you did in the past. You were the only one to listen
to me when I was sad or happy, and you always
took the time to listen to me. I do not have a sister,
no one to talk to as I used to talk to you because
you did listen to me and spend time with me. If I
speak to others about my feelings, they tease me
and make fun of me; no one is like you, and your
classmates are visiting us very often. They also
cry a lot. Nikalette, you should know that your
friends are missing you too a lot, they come all the
time to talk to us and cry with us.

Nikalette, since you died, it is extremely hard
on mom, too; she cries a lot and always goes to the
cemetery to pray to you. Everybody in the family

is sad, a lot of crying, including your classmates, family, and friends. We feel better when we go to church, and we have deep faith in God. I know he is taking care of us, but I will always try to be strong like you and continue with school. I am on the honor roll now. I am going for confirmation program and Bible classes. I will be successful because you encouraged me to do good in school and sports. I always said my prayers daily. I love you very much, and you are always with me. I miss you a lot. It is a good thing I have a lot of pictures of you and excellent memories of you to keep me company. I love you, and I miss you a lot. I think about you every day.

Angelina, your younger sister

A dear family friend, whom we considered part of our family, wrote this note about Nikalette:

It is hard for me to pick just one memory to share of Nikalette, I have so many to choose from, and for me, words just do not seem adequate. Instead, I would like to try to explain who Nikalette was to me. From the first day I met her, she adopted me into her family and her heart. I had no choice in the matter. She was the daughter I never had.

Nikalette was only three months older than my son Camiel and so for most of their lives they went to school together and grew up together. I got to enjoy every milestone twice. She always told everybody that I was her aunt. I was a disciplinarian in her life and I do not think she had ever been in time-out or the corner until she met me, but instead of rebelling against that, she embraced it and strived to make me proud every step of the way.

I spent countless hours with Nikalette curling and braiding her hair for all occasions, giving her rides to events, helping her with her homework and school projects. I even taught her how to dance when she was little. Even back then, she tried to lead as if she just did not understand how to follow.

She would come to me for advice about anything and everything. She would video chat to choose which outfit or shoes were the best for whatever the occasion, or a phone call about how she wanted to keep her friend from self-harming. She really cared about people and wanted to help them love themselves and help them know they could reach their goals if they just did not give up.

Nikalette was so full of life and had so much to give—a very compassionate and spiritual young girl. She wanted to be able to do all the things other teenagers were doing, even when her mother would warn her that she was not able to. Nikalette was stubborn and refused to let her epilepsy hold her back. She wanted to live life to the fullest, and she did. She would get out there, join things, and immerse herself in giving back to those around her.

There was never a time that I did not see her express her absolute gratitude to those who helped her or gave back to her. For example, she would always refuse to tell me what she wanted for a birthday gift because she said that I did enough for her every day and did not need to buy her a gift, yet she would always make sure she got me a gift for my birthday.

Nikalette might have been a bit of a sassy-mouthed diva, but she was so much more than that. In addition, Nikalette had a thirst for knowledge, which made her curious about everything. She was a bit naive, but she did not let it stop her from asking question after question.

I always knew when she was about to blurt out some random bizarre, crazy question because she would start twirling my hair and give me with this look as if she was thinking of the best way to ask it. The gears were turning in her head, and yet I was always surprised by the audaciousness once the question was asked. She did not just laugh all the time. She would also make others around her laugh because she would be so full of mirth and joy, it was contagious.

She was also a great listener and would listen to other people's problems as well. In addition, she absolutely loved babies and little children. She was always playing with them or wanting to hold them. I have two young nieces, and she was forever carrying them around or sitting them on her lap. She would always tell me how one day, when she will be married, she would have a bunch of beautiful mixed babies with colored eyes. I would laugh at her and shake my head because this always led to her asking me how to get them to have blue eyes like mine. One of the last conversations she had with me was at my house; while she was laying across my bed, she asked me if I would cry at her funeral. I told her that she was not allowed to die before me and that she damn well better come to my funeral and bring all her friends because none of mine would be there.

I was just trying to tease her and lighten the mood because I had no idea where that question came from, but then I got serious and I told her that of course I would cry. That I would be beyond devastated and there would be no consoling me. That she would be missed and loved by everybody, not just me, and that I pray I never have to see the day. She just nodded her head yes, that she understood and had her answer and then she promised me she would go to my funeral and bring all her friends. I mention this because it was literally a few weeks before she passed that she asked me this. Nikalette just had a feeling; she knew it was going to be her time. She is looking down on us all and sees how much she is absolutely loved and missed, and I know she is looking out for us.

Nikki Amber Pate

These notes are from Nikalette's mother Sandra Edith Simental Batten, given to me very recently so that I could publish them in this book.

My mother has been asking me for several months to write about my experience with my daughter Nikalette. It has been extremely difficult to do. Every time I hesitate.

It has been over a year, and I still feel like I am living a dream, a very painful situation. I am living a nightmare. Wishing it was a dream that I could wake up from. I miss her so very much every single moment of every day. Whenever I started to write about her, or would mention memories of her, and I would cry and cry for hours. My daughter was special. She was a mini-me, although she never liked that. I would tell her so, but I knew that deep down she did like it. Nikalette had a beautiful personality, a big bright smile, luxurious long, brown, wavy hair, her beautiful light brown eyes, and her tan skin tone. She had her father's Puerto Rican attitude and was strong-minded. Nikalette was determined to be a leader. Nikalette's father died when she was not even a year old, and she never got to make memories with him. But her father was crazy about her.

I used to tell her, "If your father had been present, he would have spoiled you very much." I do regret not telling her more stories about him. She felt very connected to him even though she did not remember him. She was extremely proud of her father and her Spanish heritage. She said I am Latina, I do speak English and Spanish, and I am bilingual. She would get upset when people would try to tell her she was not Puerto Rican since she was only half. She wanted to represent her father in everything she did so that he could be proud of her and her achievements in school and sports.

Now I realize how much she was missing him in her life and remember how much she wanted to do her best for him to be proud of her, even though her father was in heaven. My daughter was beautiful inside and out. She was caring, compassionate, and determined to be successful with any task she set forth to do, including academics, sports, music, and community work. Nikalette was an extremely spiritual girl who did her prayers every day with her grandmother, my mother, and she subscribed to an app on her phone to receive daily Bible scriptures as well. We did not know that until after she went to heaven. Nikalette loved God and had deep faith in Jesus Christ.

One month before she died, she went to see her siblings on her father's side in Tampa, Florida. He had two older sons and two daughters, Juni, Janessa, Cesar, and Raquel. I am glad that she visited them because she had a good time and got to know them better. She became remarkably close to them and to her nieces as well. Nikalette loved children very much and enjoyed being an aunt to her older sister's two daughters. She loved her two nieces, one of them was about five years old and the baby was a few months.

Nikalette wanted to become a pediatric neurologist. She admired her doctors, Dr. Nadia and Dr. Farha Tokarz, her pediatrician and her neurologist. Those two women were influential in her life. Nikalette wanted to attend Loyola University in Chicago, Illinois, to study medicine. She took a tour of Loyola in her junior year and was extremely excited that day when she came home. She said, "I found the university for medical school!"

I miss my daughter very much, but I know one day I will be reunited with my baby girl forever in heaven when God calls me to be in his kingdom. I am still grieving her and will continue to grieve, even if less often with time, for my baby girl. Nikalette never allowed her diagnosis as epileptic to stop her from doing anything. She was a true warrior princess who battled her epilepsy every day. She would not allow herself to get enough rest because she just wanted a normal teenage life.

Nikalette wanted to accomplish so many things in life that she made me extremely nervous at times because she did not want to stop school activities, was eager to learn, and wanted to help her fellow classmates, all while continuing her academic goals. She excelled in her studies and was going to graduate early from high school. I constantly worried because of the nocturnal seizures, the grand mal seizures, that only happened during her sleep. Sometimes her face would turn blue from not being able to breathe. She would get body convulsions and mouth secretions only during the night in her sleep. However, she wanted to live a normal life.

Nikalette was truly a warrior princess who battled her epilepsy by doing a lot for other people in need. I do have many regrets; maybe if we would have prayed harder together with Nikalette, God would have healed her from epilepsy. I miss her so much. Every day we went out for coffee or went to stores to buy supplies for school projects. I miss the times when she asked me to buy clothes and shoes.

I think that maybe because she had no father in her life and because of her strong faith in God, she matured fast. Nikalette was very friendly and compassionate, always trying to help her classmates who were lonely or having problems at school. She helped so many students to resolve so many problems. Nikalette became immensely popular with all her classmates of different races, genders, and religions at Aurora West High School. She was very well accepted and respected in any group that she interacted with. With her lovely personality, my baby was extra special. She was mini-me but more perfect than me—she was a very spiritual girl. She did everything with passion and a good attitude. I gave a freedom and trust to Nikalette to go to school events, parties with friends, and sports. She was a cheerleader and played all sports for more than twelve years: soccer, volleyball, and football. She was so serious about everything. She was very successful with academics, sports, religion, and community volunteer work. I did admire her; she had so much drive. She was the joy of the family with a lot of energy and a good attitude—an extraordinary girl with so many talents. And all the people that she encountered loved my girl. She did power lifts at the gym five times a week. I was concerned for her health, but I would still give her the freedom to go to school events, party with her friends, and be involved in all of her sports activities. She was a cheerleader, volleyball player, and soccer player for many years.

Nikalette had a lot of friends, a big family, and a big heart. She loved everybody, and she was happy and busy, very disciplined in the pursuit of any task that she endeavored. I never allowed her to date any boys because I wanted her to be focused on school. I always told her, "The boys are a distraction; focus on school. One day, when you go to college, you will find a boyfriend in college, where people will be more mature." However, Nikalette did have a boyfriend at school for two months before she died. He is from an exceptionally good family, and he is also an extremely popular sports person, just like she was.

The day that she went to the Lord, she'd had a very stressful day. She found out that she did not make the soccer team, which hurt her deeply. She also was told by her friend that her boyfriend was seen with another girl. She was heartbroken by this but did not mention it to any of us in her family. She was also going through a lot of stress at school because of a presentation she had to give on top of two tests as well. Her favorite uncle, Jose Pucho, her father's youngest brother, had had an accident, and she was worried about him as well. With all of this stress, Nikalette's brain could not handle it and triggered the fatal seizure that took her life. I regret I was not home that night. I went to work, so I was not able to be there when she was having the grand mal seizure and she was dying. Her heart was broken, and the stressed brain was the cause of her death.

But I know that I will see her again and that, at least now, she is free of seizures. Nikalette would pray and pray every day, asking God to stop the grand mal seizures. I believe he did listen to Nikalette, but God took her with Him to His kingdom for eternal life so that she would no longer suffer from epilepsy. Today my life is empty without her, but I feel her presence. I know she is our angel and watches over her siblings and me. She always gives me signs to let me know she is here with me. God knew that we needed a special angel to get through the rest of our days. I know that some people do not believe in a higher being and the grace of God, but I can feel it because I trust the Lord Jesus Christ.

The day before Nikalette passed, she had worked on a special project at school, painting a heart on a shirt even though her classmates all painted something different. I know that shirt was for me, her family, and her friends.

She wanted to be perfect with everything she put her mind to. She painted a beautiful heart, it was well done, painted with love. It was her way to say "good-bye, but my love always will be with all of you."

After Nikalette died, her chemistry teacher Ms. Smith brought me the shirt with the heart on it. The shirt is so pretty. I see the heart and it reminds me of her. Even though she is not physically here with us, her spirit is. The heart on the shirt is the reason we bought her tombstone in the shape of a heart, and we added Our Lady of Guadalupe because Nikalette and her father Ramon were devoted to the Virgin. She was very attached to Virgin Guadalupe ever since she visited Mexico City.

Nikalette is now our angel and will forever be an incredibly lovely daughter. I thank God for everything, and I do have a strong faith in God. I would not be here without my faith and without God. I do not want to exist with no faith. I want all the readers of this book to know that having faith is immensely powerful. God will bring us home one day, because all of us eventually will die. But we need to be good and confess to Jesus Christ as our Savior so that we may go to heaven with Him. God calls us when He needs us in His kingdom. He needed Nikalette there, and that is why He took her peacefully. We must prepare for our last home in heaven because the day will come.

I met a wonderful man a couple of months before Nikalette died. He has been a huge support to my family and me throughout this time, after twelve years of raising my four children with only my parents' extreme support. I think Nikalette might have known that she was going to go be with the Lord and her father, Ramon. She wanted to make sure I would be ok, and that is why this man has come into my life in my greatest time of need.

Nikalette's legacy will be forever. She touched the lives of so many friends and classmates, most of them still grieving with us. They come to visit us often to cry or to talk about all their memories with my daughter. A few of her classmates and friends, including myself, even have her name tattooed on our skin. Nikalette's name is on my wrist. I know that she loves that her friend did that too. And one of her best friends just had a baby sister, and her mother named her Nikalette.

My oldest son is now a father and wanted to have a girl so that he could name her after Nikalette as well. He had a boy instead and named him Milton. He was due around Nikalette's birthday, but he came early. He was born on February 16, 2020. He is healthy and beautiful, with loving parents.

Our family, friends, and her classmates visited us often for dinner, for prayers, or just to talk about memories of Nikalette. It's been incredibly sad to see that several friends are not doing well at school or in their personal lives. We all are grieving together as a family and community. This book that my mother is preparing for Nikalette will be a memory of her to those who knew her well. Nikalette would want the readers to know that as long as you have God in your life and put Him first above all things, then all of your worries will be taken care of one day.

One of Nikalette's favorite quotes from the Bible was Matthew 19:26: "for God all things are possible." Plans never happened; the golden years we never knew. We bury dreams, but in heaven, these dreams will be true. As Acts 3:21 reminds us, God has promised an eternal life "whom heaven must receive until the times of universal resto-

ration of which God spoke through the mouth of his holy prophets from of old."

Finally, death seems to take so much. We bury not just a body but the degrees of school. What was promised never happened. The dreams of my daughter included one day becoming a doctor. We never saw that in life, but in heaven, those dreams will come true. Let the promise of heaven change you from mindful to hopeful, from dwellers in the land of good-bye to the heaven of hello. God has promised a restoration of all.

I know one day I will be reunited with my baby girl. My heart will once again be filled with happiness and joy. Until then, I will continue my journey on this earth to give testimony regarding the life of Nikalette, the warrior princess who battled epilepsy, and her deep faith in God.

She touched so many people in her short life even though she suffered a lot with grand mal seizures. Now she is our pure, beautiful guardian angel. Anyone in heaven, whether your grandpa, your aunt, your child, or any family member, is waiting for the day when God s family is back together; shouldn't we do the same?

ALL the gatherings with Nikalette's family, school friends, and church leaders were extremely beneficial for all of us during the grieving pro-

cess, first we had the Christian music and prayers very similar with any church service or mass, then they read poems, letters. And they spoke about Nikalette's qualities. With all those poems and letters you the reader would have a better picture of my loving granddaughter, every May 10 we have a very similar meeting at the cemetery.

Sandy Simental Batten

CHAPTER 17

Nikalette's Special Celebration

Nikalette's Life Celebration: A Year After She Went to Heaven

Nikalette's memorial service was held at her gravesite on May 10, 2019. We brought pink and red roses, played Christian music, and shared Bible readings along with reflections, poems, and prayers. Her classmates spoke with gratitude about their positive experiences with Nikalette.

We all visited the cemetery. Leading us for prayer, scripture readings, and reflections were Monsignor Robert Willhite and Luis Patiño, a deacon from Saint Rita of Cascia Church in Aurora. They both gave Holy Bible readings with reflections. One of the readings was John 14:1–6:

"Do not let your hearts be troubled. You have faith in God; have faith also in me. In my Father's house there are many dwelling places. If there were not, would I have told you that I am going to prepare a place for you? And if I go and prepare a place for you, I will come back again and take you to myself, so that where I am you also may be. Where I am going you know the way." Thomas said to him, "Master, we do not know where you are going; how can we know the way?" Jesus said to him, "I am the way, the truth, and the life. No one comes to the father except through me."

Reflecting on that reading was helpful for me and for others. It reminded us that to have faith in our Lord Jesus Christ is accepting the departure of our loved ones, because our Lord is in control of our lives.

The turnout at the memorial service was terrific. More than 150 people attended this ceremony. We felt Nikalette's spirit and the Holy Spirit's presence everywhere. The Christian songs at her gravesite precipitated our emotions; we could not stop crying, remembering Nikalette. This ceremony was beneficial for the grieving. We all cried and prayed together, and her classmates and friends shared many stories about Nikalette.

The religious ceremony lasted forty-five minutes. Several classmates spoke about Nikalette's attitude and care for others. Then suddenly the sun came out of the clouds, and we felt both the power of the Holy Spirit and Nikalette's presence. One of her friends took a picture, which shows a cross reflecting over Nikalette's gravesite from the light of the sky. Everyone made a loud surprised noise, then was quiet. It was a cloudy day, but suddenly the sun was out. All become calm and serene. It was a very emotional and beautiful experience. Most of us had tears in our eyes, crying for our princess.

The celebration of Nikalette's life, on this first anniversary, continued at the Prestbury Clubhouse. Nikalette's family, friends, and classmates from Aurora West High School all gathered for a dinner reception. Several students spoke about Nikalette: how much they miss her and her smile, how she was able to help them with anything from academics to exercise. They shared beautiful memories, including praying together before a test. All those stories were beneficial for our healing process and for our grieving as a community.

The service was led by Nikalette's mother, Sandy. She diligently prepared and organized everything for this celebration. Everyone who attended was touched in so many ways. We all had tears in our eyes. How blessed we were to have Nikalette in our lives. Sandy bought T-shirts with Nikalette's picture on them, and a lot of the students wear them for any occasion honoring Nikalette.

Another way for us to remember my granddaughter is the custom rosary made by Marian Memories, which was handcrafted from rose petals taken from her funeral arrangement.

"And he said to them, thus it written that the Messiah would suffer and rise from the dead on the third day and that repentance, for the forgiveness of sins, would be preached in his name to all nations, beginning from Jerusalem."
Luke 24:46–47

CHAPTER 18

Growing Close to God: A Nurse's Faith

I hope Nikalette's life will motivate others who read this book to develop a close relationship with our Creator. Whether you believe in God or only know Him from a distance, my granddaughter's life can inspire you. Our Lord has a love for everyone unconditionally. It does not matter where you have been or what you are facing now, whether that's an illness affecting your body or mind, unemployment, divorce, loneliness, the loss of a loved one, family problems, drugs, COVID-19, or any other ugly experience you might be dealing with right now. I ask you, the reader, to put everything in our Lord's hands with faith and prayers. He will turn things around for the good, just as He is helping us as a family.

Deep in your soul is God. He wants you to give everything to Him. Unload your problems and illness to

Him. He will help you as He is helping me go through any difficult time. He has been with me in other stressful situations in the past, with my family and my patients. In God's hands, we can survive anything. He will help you too. You have to open yourself to the Lord to receive His Grace. He listens to our prayers, and our requests may bring pain relief or even a cure for a mental or physical problem. We do not see Him, but we can feel His presence, as Nikalette thought as well. As Mark 11:24 reminds us: "Therefore I tell you, all that you ask for in prayer, believe that you will receive it and it shall be yours."

We do not know when God will be calling us home as he called my granddaughter at the age of seventeen. Reflection is a simple way to pray to God, and you will receive such peace with yourself. It does not matter who you are or where you have been; we all need to believe in our Creator.

We are born to die. All of us are going to die one day. We do not know when, but no one will live here forever. Our memories, life trajectory, and input into this life will stay with our families and friends. The question is how we want to be remembered.

It does not matter where you are at present with spirituality, religion, or beliefs in life. We are in charge of our lives in the way we decide to live, making good or bad decisions, and we face the consequences. But always remember: God is our Creator who loves all of us. I am telling you; God loves you.

What matters is our faith. A believing person will have more peace in life and death. It would be beneficial to have a religion and a good support system from family, church, or a community. It is essential to belong to a church group. You will meet good friends who can help you in good times and bad times, as I experienced with the sudden loss of Nikalette. We can accomplish so many things in life; we need to connect with our Lord to have a peaceful, happy, and successful life. With repentance, we may go to heaven and transcend to the other life. Who knows? In our next life, we do not know if heaven is for us; no one knows where our spirit will go after death.

Our bodies will be buried in the cemetery or will be cremated. Death can happen anytime, but we all will go through it. We do not want to go, and we do not want our loved ones to die either, but this is part of life. Now, the very uncertain times around the world with this pandemic affecting us in all aspects—physical, mental, social, and economical—this time we are living is dangerous. There may be other viruses, climate changes, and war. Jesus came to free us from anything.

God is in control. God will be calling us home as he called my granddaughter. We do not like to discuss anything regarding death. It is uncomfortable to plan for the end of life. But we can prepare for eternal life by accepting the Lord in our hearts, by practicing our faith and joining a church, even in a rural or small town. It does not matter what you call Him. The important thing is that you have faith in Him.

Even if you have no church, you can still read the Bible and other religious books and have a routine to pray or speak to God daily. He will lead you in the right direction. Now with technology, it is easier. I used the internet, YouTube, and Facebook when the church in my town was closed from March through July 2020 due to the pandemic. You can also learn religion. I am optimistic that you will be happier.

Becoming wealthy or having power is not making us happy: we can have everything but still feel empty. When we become close to God, we are comfortable and able to resolve conflicts and problems with more wisdom. As deep as your faith is, you will receive grace from God, as my granddaughter did. God is good to all of us who trust Him. I do not want to live my life empty, not trusting God, or not having strong faith. I would not be able to survive. I would not be happy. That is my personal belief, and I trust Jesus Christ.

I do recall once working on a medical mission trip to another country. I was exhausted from working long hours in the hospital, but the next day, I still traveled out of the United States to take care of poor and sick patients. The medical and nursing team prayed together each morning before and each evening after a long shift. I was praying that I would function well as a nurse. I was exhausted from working so many shifts. God did help me because I performed my job well. I had a lot of energy to take care of patients. I made my career as a clinical nurse, plus I had an opportunity to work with many people from different countries and states. The medical missionaries, a large group of people from the United States, were primarily doctors, nurses, a few dentists, and others volunteer for construction. We took care of more than one thousand patients in ten days. We did an excellent job working as a team doing everything from surgical procedures to staffing outpatient clinics, and the outcome was good. It was a very spiritual team and a fascinating experience.

I returned home, and I was pleased with the satisfaction, peace, energy, and beautiful feeling that we had generated during our medical mission. I believe this is how our Lord works with us. I was an instrument of Him helping sick and poor people. God took care of my family at home while I did work as a nurse on a mission trip to another country.

Holistic nursing care was provided at most hospitals and clinics that I worked at, which benefitted patients in many ways. It included spiritual, physical, social, and psychological care twenty-four hours a day, which is essential to maintaining our health. The Bible was in each patient's room, and pastoral care and a chapel for Mass or other religious services were provided to patients and families. They were satisfied with the patient care that we provided.

However, I do respect any religion or other beliefs. Any person who already has a deep faith should continue praying for a healthy world. We all need each other, especially now with this COVID-19 pandemic. Are we going to have other viruses or other global problems? God, please help us. We need to get close to God for our health; as Nikalette stated, "Now before our opportunity is gone, we need to have faith."

Encouragement: Practicing Nursing Care with Faith

In my experience as a Registered nurse, I gained a lot of knowledge about the nursing profession. I've worked in so many different clinical settings, from severely ill patients to rehabilitation, and in both medical and surgical units. I loved my job tremendously. I worked for various hospitals and nursing homes as well as home health care, nursing agency and teaching nursing students. To improve patient care, I researched nationally and presented national and internationally on health topics. I love my nursing profession.

I include spiritual care when requested by the patient, because I believe we all need holistic care as part of nursing care along with physical, emotional, social, and recreational attention. That means healing the mind, body, and soul of the individual and integrating the principles and the modalities of holistic healing into daily life and clinical practice: self-care, self-responsibility, spirituality, and reflection in their lives.

I helped many terminally ill patients die from cancer or other acute illnesses. Many of them were afraid, sick, in acute pain, with a high anxiety level, and depressed from being ill for a long time. They were , at times, with no family around them. They were very lonely. Several patients stayed in the hospital for more than a year on different floors with multiple medical problems from intensive care to regular medical and surgical floors. A few of them did not have a place to go after discharge. Some had no one to help them at home, no significant others. The difference was that if they had a deep, strong faith in God, they all died very peacefully, as my Nikalette died in her sleep.

Other patients recuperated with no complications, only through faith in our Creator, even with no significant others, other patients no family only a community or church support system. I cared for patients who had no support system and no faith in God. They suffered more when they were hospitalized or when they were dying. No one was with them at that time, only the hospital staff. Today we have cases similar due to this pandemic. My daughter Sandy is working with COVID-19 patients, and I am praying daily for all the healthcare providers, first responders, caregivers and patients. And for all people working in any clinical setting. No visitors are allowed at the hospital for those patients who are in isolation. Most of the time, we were only able to call the hospital chaplain who assisted those patients in dying peacefully.

For the majority of the time, nursing staff is the first line of workers with patients in hospitals. They serve as a nurse and even as a pastor to pray for those patients. But all personnel are essential, whether they're housekeepers, clerks, dieticians, doctors, nurses, respiratory therapists, and other employees of the hospital and clinics. They deserve a lot of respect for their magnificent job, and compassion to take care of very sick patients and have respect for all patients, families, and staff. Especially considering the potential that they may also become ill.

When it was requested by the patient or patient's family, I would pray with them. Several patients told me they regretted not knowing the Lord until they were close to death. Other patients told me they were incredibly lonely. Other patients said that they had an opportunity to form a family with a spouse and children, but they refused. They said they had not wanted any responsibilities later in life. They were very lonely and sick. They said that they regretted their choice. They were rich with all the material things, but it did not make them happy until they found God at the hospital when they were so sick or close to death.

At times, we experience emptiness in us for different reasons. To attempt to remain young, we turn to vain, selfish, material things, like plastic surgery. The materials things all come and go; youth and good looks, with the aging process, will decline. Nothing will make us happy without our spiritual life connected to our Lord Jesus Christ the Creator. He is the only one who can make us happy and provides all of us with His grace, as He offered to Nikalette. And He can help us to resolve conflicts and problems peacefully with more wisdom. Our faith allows us to see what unseen is, like paradise, like eternal life with our Lord and loved ones who have already departed from this temporal life.

It does not matter what you want to call him: Our Creator, Our Lord, Jesus Christ, Allah. The important thing is that we have our faith to be sustained in any crisis. I take this opportunity to invite all of you who are reading this book to become active and practice your faith by joining a church or religious community. Our body needs holistic care and spiritual friends to deal with tragedies in life.

Overall, we all need to be prepared to meet God as Nikalette was. Trust God to enhance your faith to be at peace with yourself and live joyfully and healthfully. For nurses around the world, I am suggesting and encouraging a prayer that I say daily for a peaceful day. As I care for my patients, the Lord is with me: "O Lord, I pray. Make my words and actions kind; it means so much for our patients, and in my hands, Lord, place Your healing touch. Let Your healing touch others. Let, Lord, your love shine through all that I do. So those in need may hear and feel your presence in Jesus Christ, amen."

I've added this chapter detailing my own experience in the nursing profession because knowing this book is Nikalette's biography, I wanted to voice my sincere beliefs in the Lord. And my passion for nursing Also, Nikalette, on her last Christmas with us, wrote a beautiful note to let me know that she would want to follow in my steps because in the future she wanted to work in hospitals and I was her role model.

Epilogue

On November 8, 2021, my grandson, Sam Anthony, Nikalette's older brother, was trying to go to work and one of his car's tires came out while he was driving. He was not able to control his car and accidentally crashed into someone's front porch. There was small damage on the house porch and he had a small laceration on his right elbow. However, his car, a 2018 Chevy Malibu, was totally destroyed. On December 21, 2021, at 11 A.M., my husband was driving in our car, a 2007 Nissan Altima, near our home in Sugar Grove; he was also in a car accident. His car was a total loss, and he was shaken and anxious, but there were no injuries. These two car accidents let me believe that our guardian angel Nikalette is watching over us and that our Lord Jesus Christ is protecting us.

Even now, people who did not know her will stop at Nikalette's grave. They stop to visit her without knowing her, and they call Nikalette the beautiful princess. Recently on Father's Day I found people visiting her; there were several members of a family with three lovely children and two parents. The children helped us to put water on Nikalette's flowers.

※

By completing this book, in both languages to honor Nikalette. I am finally accepting the plan of God. We will be able to see Nikalette again when our Lord Jesus Christ calls us into His presence one day. It fills me with joy to pass on to eternal life because I am positive that Nikalette is in heaven and I know that I will see my granddaughter again one day. It serves as a consolation for me and the rest of her family and friends. Nikalette is not suffering from epilepsy anymore.

Our family, the Aurora community, and I accept that this separation is only temporary, even though it has been painful and difficult. Things are now feeling better. Our deep faith sustains us, knowing that we all are born with Christ, live with Christ, and die with Christ. God is more significant than all things in this world, so we should not fear. I have been enormously blessed to know that I did my best to guide, love, and assist Nikalette with any of her needs. One of the main reasons I wanted to publish her book is to help others who have epilepsy and their families.

Remember John 11:25: "Jesus told her, 'I am the resurrection and the life; whoever believes in me, even if he dies, will live.'"

I chose to write Nikalette's biography, a true story reflecting her life, experiences, achievements, and deep love for God and others, because I am highly optimistic that my experience and knowledge would benefit all of you who read this book.

A reminder of the subjects covered in this book honoring Nikalette:

- The biography of our Nikalette
- Yabucoa Puerto Rican first Princess 2017–2018.
- Awareness of epilepsy and grief.
- Inspiration to develop firm faith in God, even with disabilities and disadvantages.
- A demonstration of our appreciation to all people who were part of Nikalette's life from birth until now.

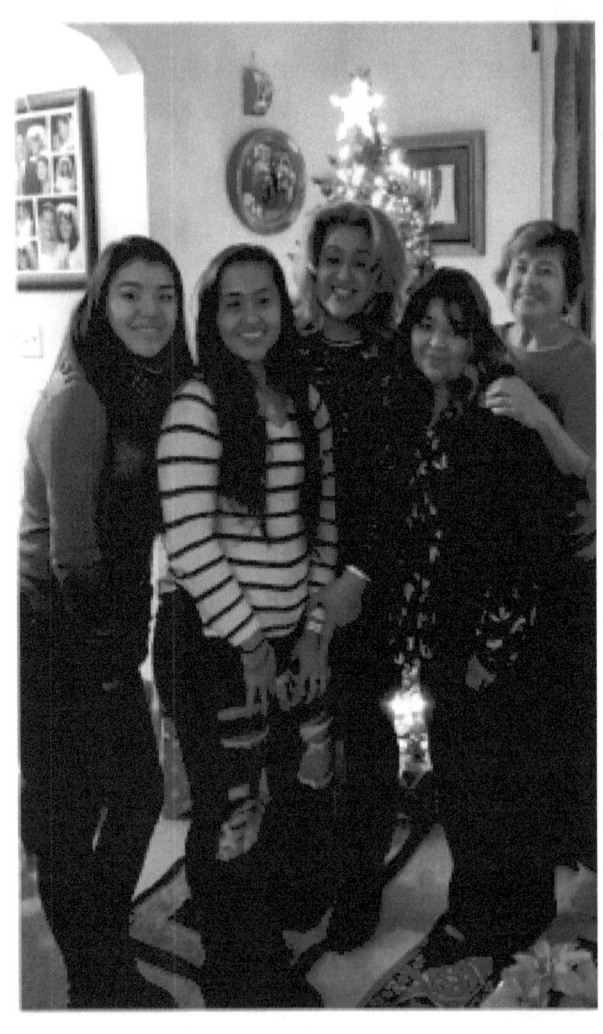

"Last Christmas with Nikalette, December 2017. She wears a
striped sweater. From left to right:
her cousin Liliana, her mother Sandy, her aunt Lily,
and me, the Grandmother.

My lovely granddaughter, the warrior princess who battled epilepsy with her big dreams for the future—her life story will be forever. One day she hoped to become a doctor to be able to treat people with epilepsy and bring them closer to God so they would be sustained by their faith. Now Nikalette is doing it through this book.

After Nikalette's death, several friends came to me and told me that they lost a family member during a seizure, mainly while in their sleep. They'd never mentioned it to me before. I never faced so many people telling me about their loved ones who died during a seizure or from complications with epilepsy. They were suffering from a lack of knowledge about epilepsy. So I've decided to share my knowledge as an experienced registered nurse and as the grandmother of Nikalette to help prevent others from potential injuries with seizures.

At times I wish I could go back to the past, even for a few moments, when I was taking care of my granddaughter. I recall her eagerness to learn and grow. I loved teaching her how to take care of patients, as well as the times we danced together to cumbias, polkas, or Spanish music or the times we went to church, to travel, or even just to take her to school. Everything is in the past, but she left a memorable mark in my heart and mind.

I hope all of you readers know that life is too fragile, and we are here temporarily and must live our day like it is the last day in this world. We need strong faith in God, a good attitude, love for others, and the ability to resolve conflicts in a peaceful manner. God is taking care of us so we can take of others as Nikalette did.

I also enjoyed reading stories and poems from Nikalette's classmates and family members that I was sure that you would like them too. They were accommodating to the grieving process. I know all of you would learn from this book regarding epilepsy, the grieving process, faith in God, and a few things from Spanish American culture. Nikalette's last assignments were included to honor and remember Nikalette. They also served us as consolation.

It is a blessing to know that my granddaughter at the age of seventeen did influence others, such as her classmates and the community of Aurora. I am confident you will be satisfied with the biography of Nikalette Simental-Rivera, the beautiful warrior princess. She battled epilepsy and all her other difficulties. But she especially had immense love for God and people. Now she is our angel in heaven, gone but not forgotten. How blessed we are to have shared Nikalette's life. Her love for our Lord Jesus Christ and all of us, her presence, contagious energy, and pleasant attitude all reflected the grace of God.

Our family, friends, and community have been more united since this sudden death of Nikalette. It changed us for the better by enhancing our faith in God and resolving conflicts an a professional manner. Our life will never be the same, but with a strong belief in our Lord Jesus Christ, we are moving forward.

God bless all you readers.

Acknowledgments

I appreciate Dr. Shirley Ambutas, APN, DNP, CCRN-K, CCNS, from Rush University Medical Center in Chicago, Illinois; Dr. Roger Rangel, MD., Mie University Hospital, Japan; Director for the Surgical/Diagnostics Clinic, Torreon, Coahuila, Mexico; Claire Perez, MRE, Bible Scripture Expert and a leader for the RITE of Christian Initiation of Adults from Saint Rita Church in Aurora, Illinois, who helped me organize this book. I thank them for their collaboration and consulting on the drafts of parts of this book.

I want to take this opportunity to give special thanks to Mr. Rafael Surillo, the mayor of Yabucoa, Puerto Rico. He provided Information about Yabucoa Puerto Rico to my granddaughter Nikalette in May 2017. Even though he had a busy day and we did not have an appointment with him, the mayor and many others in Yabucoa were extremely helpful and provided literature regarding the town's history. Nikalette was able to write her research paper, adding information about her own experience in Yabucoa, Puerto Rico. Also, thanks to the police department of Yabucoa, Puerto Rico, and a special thanks to the police officer, Mr. Pablo Prico Ortiz, who gave us a tour of the city and its surroundings.

With appreciation to the leaders and directors of the Aurora Puerto Rican Cultural Council, Miss Iris Miller, Ms. Mirna Rivera, and their committee members. There are not enough words to express our sincere appreciation to all family members, friends, students, teachers, and the community of Aurora, Illinois, for the overwhelming sympathy, love, and support during this challenging time for all of us. In the cemetery, Nikalette has fresh flowers and balloons. Her classmates, friends, and families still visit her at the cemetery.

We appreciate the mayor, Mr. Richard C. Irwin, for his participation and collaboration in preserving and maintaining Spanish Latino American Culture in Aurora, Illinois.

I am extremely appreciative of Mrs. Sheila McQuade, Nikalette's HOSA English teacher; Miss Smith, her chemistry teacher; and all the other teachers and staff from Aurora West High School for the memorial service to honor Nikalette Simental-Rivera. We thank them for their dedication to all their students.

Thanks to Saint Rita of Cascia Church in Aurora, Illinois; Father Oscar Cortes, Father Gerardo Manuel Gomez, and Rev. Msgr Robert Willhite; the deacons, staff, pastors, and friends from Calvary Temple, Naperville, Illinois. All our community thanks you for all the spiritual support and religious education provided to Nikalette and our family.

I would also like to thank my parents, Jose and Guadalupe Rangel, for giving me the fantastic values of religion, education, family, and community work. My brothers and sisters in blood and in Christ and extended family members, friends, and teachers serve me as role models and mentors. You've shown love and motivated me to reach my professional goals and maintain unity in my family, placing God first in our lives. Thanks to the Simental family for the spiritual support and wisdom provided to us.

I am thankful to God that I strongly believe in Jesus Christ as my Savior. He brought me to the best country globally, the United States of America. A better life and allowing me to travel around the world as a missionary nurse for several medical trips and for vacations provided me the opportunity to write this book, which took three years off and on to complete. And thanks lastly to my husband, Juan, and adult children and their families, for the encouragement and for standing by me through this situation.

I also offer my sincere appreciation for your time to read this story. Nikalette's family and friends cherish the beautiful moments we had with our warrior princess. We hope you found her life story spiritual, engaging, and full of love, giving you the inspiration to continue in life, even with any disadvantage, pain, or crises you may face.

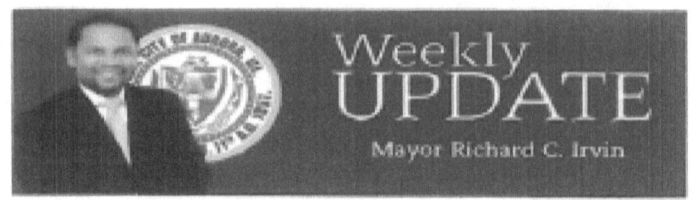

Monday, July 30, 2018

In the Spotlight

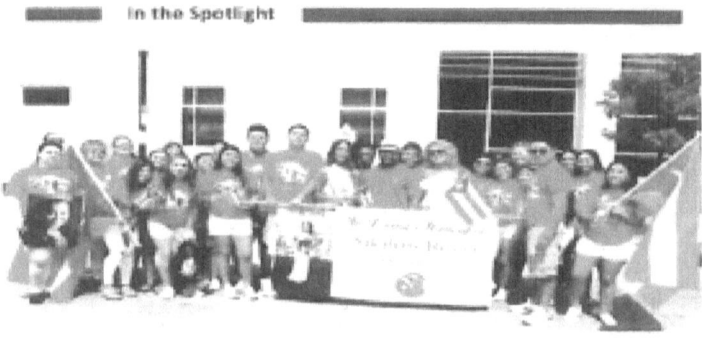

IN LOVING MEMORY OF NIKALETTE RIVERA
More than 100 family and friends formed a special unit in the Puerto Rican Heritage Parade in memory of Nikalette Rivera. The 17 year-old First Princess of the Aurora Puerto Rican Cultural Council, Nikalette

On July 29, 2018, the president of the Aurora Puerto Rican Cultural Council, Iris Miller, began the Puerto Rico parade with gratitude to our town Aurora Illinois. One section of the speech was to honor the memory of Nikalette Simental Rivera, our Yabucoa Puerto Rican Princess 2017–2018. More than one hundred family, students and friends attended the parade section to honor the memory of Nikalette. I offer my thanks to the leaders, teachers, students, friends, and Nikalette's family members who participated in this event. All the classmates and friends wore white shorts and red T-shirts with Nikalette's picture that day, which was also Nikalette's father's birthday.

I also offer appreciation to all of you who attended the gatherings to remember Nikalette on May 10, 2019, and May 10, 2020, and the students, families, and friends who came to our home and visited Nikalette's gravesite. We all grieved together as a community. The Simental and Rivera families are thankful for your kindness, support, and understanding during that period of pain following the sudden death of our warrior princess, Nikalette Simental-Rivera

References

Castro Vargas, Luis Fernando. "Muerte súbita e inesperada en la epilepsia (sudep)." *Medicina Legal de Costa Rica*, 30(2) (Septiembre 2013): 93-105. http://www.scielo.sa.cr/scielo.php?script=sci_arttext&pid=S1409-00152013000200011&lng=en&tlng=es.

Clark, Damian and Kate Riney. "A population-based postmortem study of sudden unexpected death in epilepsy." *Journal of Clinical Neuroscience*, Volume 23 (2016): 58-62. https://doi.org/10.1016/j.jocn.2015.04.027.

Devinsky, Orrin. "Sudden, Unexpected Death in Epilepsy." *The New England Journal of Medicine*, Volume 34 (November 10, 2011): 1801–1811. https://doi.org/10.1056/NEJMra1010481

Epilepsy Foundation. https://www.epilepsy.com. Accessed November 20, 2022.

Helpline Epilepsy. 1-800-332-1000.

Epilepsy Society. "Seizure Types." Accessed April 11, 2022. https://epilepsysociety.org.uk/about-epilepsy/epileptic-seizures/seizure-types

Hickey, Joanne V., *The Clinical Practice of Neurological and Neurosurgical Nursing*. 4th ed. Philadelphia: Lippincott-Raven Publishers, 1997.

Maguire M.J., Jackson C.F., Marson A.G., Nevitt S.J. "Treatments for the prevention of Sudden Unexpected Death in Epilepsy (SUDEP)." *Cochrane Database Syst. Rev.* 2020;4:CD011792. https://doi.org/10.1002/14651858.CD011792.pub3.

National Institute of Neurological Disorders and Stroke. *The Epilepsies and Seizures: Hope Through Research*. Bethesda, MD: National Institutes of Health, n.d. https://www.ninds.nih.gov/health-information/patient-caregiver-education/hope-through-research/epilepsies-and-seizures-hope-through-research.

Nursing.com. "Nursing Care Plan (NCP) for Seizures." https://nursing.com/lesson/nursing-care-plan-for-seizures.

Sperling, Michael R. "Sudden Unexplained Death in Epilepsy." *Epilepsy Currents* 1,1 (September 2001): 21–23. https://doi.org/10.1046/j.1535-7597.2001.00012.x

Taipei Times. "Doctor puts forward new theory about Bruce Lee's death." February 26, 2006. https://www.taipeitimes.com/News/world/archives/2006/02/26/2003294744

Topiramate: New Advances in the Treatment of Epilepsy. Vol 37, (2016): Supplement 2.